Library of
Davidson College

The People's Remedy

The People's Remedy

Health Care in
El Salvador's War of Liberation
by Francisco Metzi

Introduction by Jenny Pearce
Translated by Jean Carroll
in collaboration with the author and Rhoda Mahler

Monthly Review Press

Copyright © 1988 by Monthly Review Press
All rights reserved

Originally published as *Por los caminos de Chalatenango: La salud en la mochila* by UCA Editores, San Salvador, El Salvador
© 1988 by UCA Editores

Library of Congress Cataloging-in-Publication Data
Metzi, Francisco, 1958–
 [Por los caminos de Chalatenango. English]
 The people's remedy: health care in El Salvador's war of liberation / by Francisco Metzi; introduction by Jenny Pearce; translated by Jean Carroll in collaboration with the author and Rhoda Mahler
 Translation of: Por los caminos de Chalatenango.
 Bibliography: p.
 ISBN 0-85345-774-3
 ISBN 0-85345-775-1 (pbk.)
 1. Medical care—El Salvador—Chalatenango. 2. El Salvador—Politics and government—1979– . I. Title
 RA 454.S2M4713 1988   88–13642
 362.1'097284—dc19   CIP

Monthly Review Press
122 West 27th Street
New York, N.Y. 10001

Manufactured in the United States of America

The people might be ignorant about some things, but they have a wisdom learned from their own reality and experience, and they know exactly how, when, and why they have been deceived throughout history. Someone once said that this country of ours is so small. . . . Yes and no. It's not so small if you walk it, and only through walking it can you see where all those real inner possibilities lie. This is the perspective that they just don't have in the United States.

—*Guillermo Manuel Ungo*

To Freddy, Willy, Luisito
　and all the rest for whom we wish we had known more
　and had been able to do things better.

To Juan and Medardo
　for the push in the right direction, and for
　their examples.

Contents

Map of El Salvador viii
Introduction by Jenny Pearce ix
Prologue 1
Map of Chalatenango 4
  1. First Steps 5
  2. The Insomniacs' Collective 10
     Interview: One Day They Asked Me If
     I Wanted to Be a Guerrilla 26
  3. Our Own Hospital 35
  4. The Lessons of El Jocotillo 42
  5. Combat in the Intestinal Zone 50
  6. Can't You See This Is an Operating Room? 57
     Interview: We Went Up into the Hills Thinking
     We'd Be Back Home in a Couple of Weeks 68
  7. Doctors Double as Architects 73
  8. Learning All We Can 80
     A Letter from Carolina 86
  9. There's No More Medicine 101
10. The Right to Eat 109
11. A Shark Attacks Our Workshop 116
12. Even If We Have to Become Monkeys Again 127
     Interview: This Is a Hospital? 150
     Interview: But I Never Lost Faith 155
13. The Battle of "Lightning" 159
14. Freddy 171
15. We're Staying Put 182
Walking Salvadoran Soil Again: An Epilogue 190
Further Reading 199
Photo section 97–100

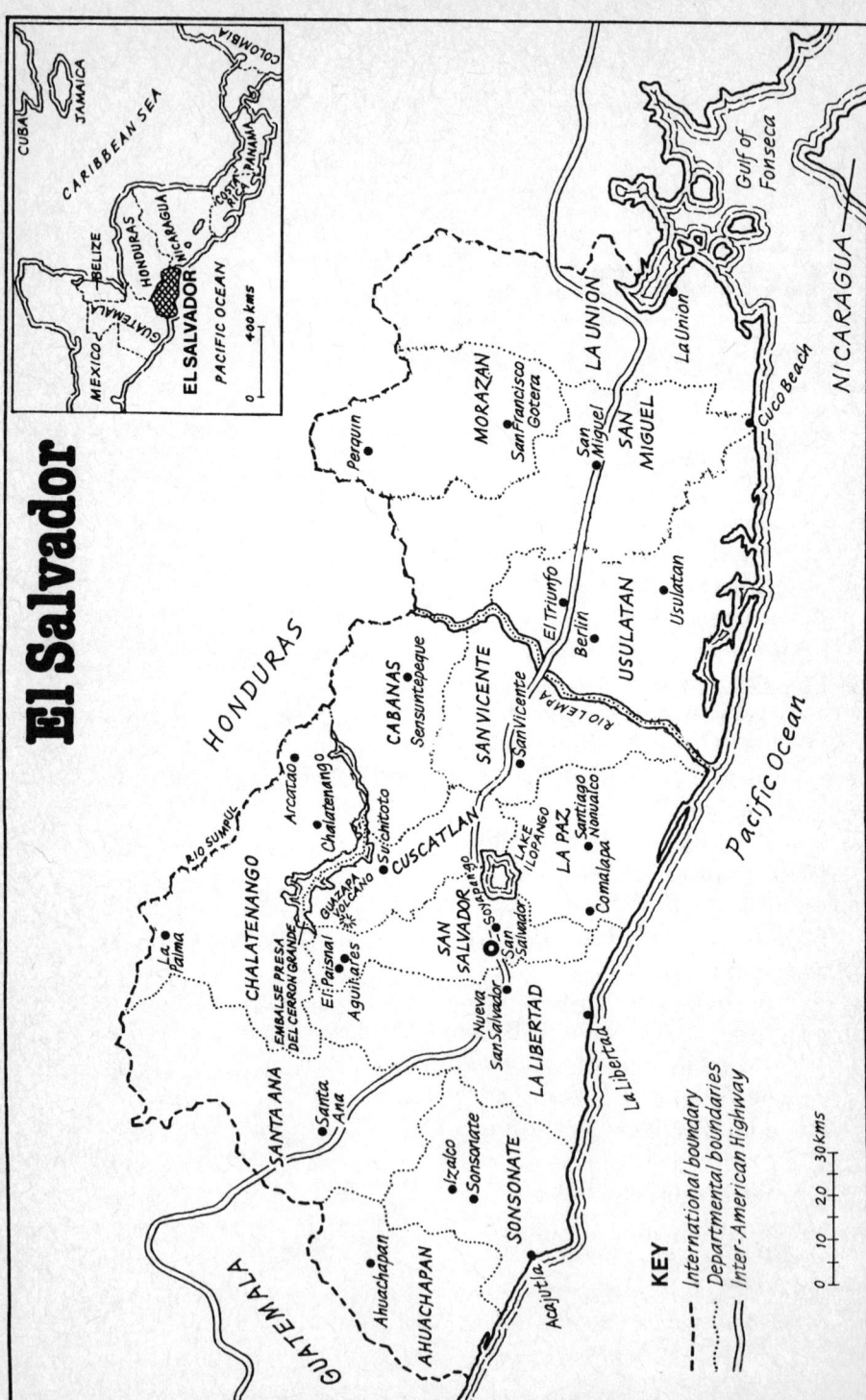

Introduction
by Jenny Pearce

Che Guevara didn't believe that armed struggle was possible in El Salvador: It would have to await the outcome of the struggles taking place in the mountainous areas of Guatemala and Nicaragua, he told the Salvadoran revolutionary leader, Salvador Cayetano Carpio, in the 1960s. A country so small and so densely populated (224 people per square mile), with no mountain or jungle hideaways, could not nurture a guerrilla army; one is never far from peasants trying to cultivate their small, eroded *parcelas* of land when walking the dirt tracks of El Salvador's countryside.

Yet El Salvador is a country now in its eighth year of guerrilla struggle, and the Faribundo Martí National Liberation Front (FMLN) is one of the most effective guerrilla forces Latin America has ever seen. It has survived through two successive terms of one of the United States' most right-wing presidents, who on coming to office in 1981 made the major theme of his foreign policy a commitment to hold back the tide of "communism" in the U.S. backyard, using El Salvador as a test case.

President Reagan has poured an estimated $3 billion in economic and military aid into El Salvador. In 1987, El Salvador became the only country since South Vietnam in which U.S. aid surpassed the government's national budget. Counterinsurgency training, U.S. military advisers, bombing campaigns, low-intensity warfare, electoral manipulation, subversion of the labor movement—the entire U.S. foreign policy arsenal has been used in El Salvador, and the United States has become a virtual parallel government in the country.

x Introduction

But despite eight years of this intense effort, four U.S. lieutenant-colonels recently concluded:

> Despite reduced numbers, the FMLN remains a formidable foe, its attacks exacerbating the deterioration of the Salvadoran economy. In a strictly tactical sense, ESAF (El Salvadoran Armed Forces) has gained the initiative. But this advantage hardly matters: observers generally concede that the FMLN—tough, competent, highly motivated—can sustain its current strategy indefinitely.*

Anyone who reads the outstanding literature of testimony and witness to come out of the Salvadoran war must gasp at the achievements of the FMLN. This book by Francisco Metzi is a fine example of this literature, and like the best of it, open and honest about the costs, the difficulties, and the mistakes involved in the guerrilla war. If you turn, for example, to the interview in this book with Emiliano (pp. 26–34), you get a flavor of the guerrilla army's humble origins. Small groups of peasants make a stick in a burlap bag look like a weapon, and with it they capture a real weapon from members of the rural vigilante organization ORDEN and pass it to the guerrillas. I heard similar stories in Chalatenango of slingshots being used to secure a weapon. The offensive of January 1981, far from being launched by a well-armed Soviet and Cuban trained guerrilla army, as Reagan told the world at the time, was conducted despite a lack of even the most basic weapons. A peasant woman who took part in the attack on the town of Chalatenango at the time told me:

> I took part in the seizure of a radio station in Chalatenango . . . at that point we didn't have any arms, we didn't have any weapons except enthusiasm. Each of us had a .38 pistol so you can see what kind of arms we had. Everyone thought it was ridiculously funny, but it was a miracle they didn't kill us all. . . . Take the provincial army HQ with a .38, yes that's suicide!**

---

*A.J. Bacavich et al., *American Military Policy in Small Wars: The Case of El Salvador*, paper delivered at the John F. Kennedy School of Government, March 22 1988.

**This and subsequent unsourced quotations are taken from J. Pearce, *Promised Land: Peasant Rebellion in Chalatenango, El Salvador* (London: Latin America Bureau, 1985).

Introduction xi

The FMLN grew in the years following the failed offensive of 1981 with the help of the enemy's conscripted peasant army, which preferred to hand over its arms and uniforms than to die in battle for an oligarchy whose sons and daughters were safely out of the way in Miami. But impressive though this military history is, it is the politics of the revolutionary process which have made El Salvador such an important example for the rest of the Third World.

* * *

Guevara and Debray's elitist and militaristic *foquista* theories of guerrilla warfare received their first serious challenge from the Forces of Popular Liberation (FPL) in El Salvador in the early 1970s. It is the FPL which came to predominate in Chalatenango, where Metzi worked as a doctor. Partly out of the necessity of the terrain, partly as a result of the political experience of its early leaders in the Salvadoran Communist Party and workers movement, and partly through lessons learned from Vietnam, the FPL opted for a strategy of combining political and military struggle. The revolution was not to be the task of a dedicated band of guerrillas, but the work of the people themselves in a prolonged popular war.

For the FPL, organizing the people in a mass movement to fight for their basic needs had a political importance in its own right; it was not just a means of raising support for the guerrillas. It is here that the FPL has departed from the strategies of most recent guerrilla movements, including those in Guatemala in the 1960s and 1970s and the FSLN in Nicaragua. Cayetano Carpio, the leader of the FPL, explained:

> We did not wish to repeat the experience of Guatemala. In Guatemala they formed support groups amongst the peasantry, not for the mass struggle, but around the logistical function, as support for the guerrillas. We, precisely because of the more integral conception that we had, and the concern not to separate ourselves from the masses (although formally we had to give up the public positions of leadership of the masses) nevertheless tried not to become detached from them.*

---

*Interview with Salvador Cayetano Carpio in M. Harnecker, *Pueblo en Armas* (Guerrero, Mexico: Universidad Autónoma de Guerrero, 1983).

This view led the FPL to respect the autonomy of the peasant organizations, the Christian Federation of Salvadoran Peasants (FECCAS) and the Union of Rural Workers (UTC), which gained widespread support in the north and east of the country, around Aguilares, Chalatenango, and San Vicente in the 1970s. In these areas, Catholic priests had begun to promote new pastoral methods, influenced by the changing theological debate in the 1960s. Most of them had no conception of the longer-term political consequences of their work. They simply wanted to see a church which served the poor instead of the state, in which a new message of justice and humanity could be debated by the people themselves.

The grass-roots communities, which were formed to enable the people to discuss this message and elect their own lay preachers, were the first rural organizations to exist independently of the state or political parties since the early 1930s. The peasants met together for the first time in a structured way; they heard that God was a just God, on the side of the poor and oppressed, and that they had the right to organize against injustice.

Peasant unionization spread rapidly in the countryside. Over the centuries, the peasants had been dispossessed of their land as one cash crop after another enriched the landed oligarchy and forced peasants into renting the poorest and least productive land. As seasonal workers on the plantations, they lived and worked in humiliating conditions. Now they organized strikes and demonstrations; occupied the Agricultural Development Bank, which had refused them credit for essential fertilizers; and in their most militant phase, took over the land which they needed to survive. Not even the fiercest repression held them back. The peasants developed their own leaders—Apolinario Serrano of FECCAS and Justo Medía of the UTC, for example—most of whom learned to read and write in the struggle. Nor did the peasant movement remain isolated in the rural areas; through the work of the FPL, it was joined with urban workers, shantytown dwellers, and students in the country's largest mass organization, the Popular Revolutionary Bloc (BPR).

This process of politicization through the people's own experience of struggle and organization helped create one of Latin America's most combative and best organized popular movements and, by the late 1970s, a genuine worker-peasant alliance. Above all, it meant that people opted to take up arms not because they were forced to or were convinced by outsiders, but because they found there was no other way of winning the means to life. The FPL won support from this peasantry because it offered the political alternative they were seeking. Its cadres worked with the peasants but did not attempt to take over their union. One peasant leader from Chalatenango told me how the work of an FPL cadre, Andrés Torres, had helped the guerrilla organization establish roots among the peasantry:

Andrés was a humble *compa*, honest and sincere. He advised us, never showing tiredness nor anger with anyone. We didn't know much about the political-military organizations at that time, we sometimes saw FPL propaganda but we had no idea that they had commandos and saw no link between what they were doing and our own organization. It was then, in 1977, that Andrés Torres was killed in Santa Tecla. And when his picture appeared in the newspaper with the letters, FPL, on the wall behind him and it turned out that he was one of the best militants of the FPL, everyone who had known him was very surprised. People's attitude began to change, many wanted to follow his example. FPL propaganda increased at this time, and its proposals tackled many of the problems we were facing in the communities. That was when we began to make contacts with the *compas* of the FPL, to find ways of getting close to the organization, and from then on our union became more politicized.

At the same time, other revolutionary groups were building strong and effective organizations in other areas. The People's Revolutionary Army (ERP) was creating an impressive military capability in Morazán, and the Armed Forces of National Resistance (FARN), with strong peasant support around Suchitoto as well as backing from workers in some of the most strategic sectors of industry, was building its own mass organization, the United Popular Action Front (FAPU).

The popular movement grew so quickly, it outpaced the capacity of the revolutionary organizations to direct it. The balance between political and military work which the FPL aimed for was difficult to maintain. In different moments in the history of the struggle, one took over the other. In these early years, it was the political work, because when it came to the formation of the FMLN out of the revolutionary groups named above and the Communist Party in 1980, there was very little in the way of a guerrilla army. The ERP had the most effective force. The FPL had to create one very rapidly, militarizing many of its popular organizations, shifting priorities from the political to the military demands of the revolution. As many as 13,000 people were killed in the last five months of 1980 during this difficult process, many of them leading cadres of the organization. And during those same months, the workers' movement in San Salvador was particularly badly hit by the repression. The newly-formed FMLN found itself a mainly rural organization by the end of the year.

The FPL had to shift its conception of the war, more so than the other revolutionary organizations. The FPL had opposed an insurrectionary strategy; it had conceived of the war as a protracted struggle, encompassing the whole country and waged by the "entire people," incorporated into it at different levels. It had never thought in terms of liberated territory, which hardly seemed appropriate or possible in El Salvador. The organization, politicization, and mobilization of the people had to compensate for the geographical disadvantages the guerrillas faced, the FPL maintained, and that would take time.

But the pace of events had quickened enormously in 1980, in the wake of the victory of the FSLN in Nicaragua. The level of popular combativity and expectation was very high. Over 200,000 people had marched in protest at the assassination of Archbishop Romero in March of that year. The pressure to launch the "final offensive" of January 1981 was overwhelming. But its subsequent failure led by necessity to a return to the strategy of prolonged war and the building of strategic rear guards—not liberated territory, for the army would always be capable of mounting invasions into any part of El Salvador, but zones of control. Chalatenango became the zone of control of the FPL. Gradually, from 1981 to 1983, the guerrillas forced the army out of the department, until it had control of twenty-eight of its thirty-three municipalities. Most secure was the eastern part of the department, and here the experiment in local democracy, the Local Popular Powers (PPLs), made its greatest advances.

The PPLs emerged in response to the necessity of organizing the population once the old authorities had fled. Food still needed to be grown and distributed, people's housing and health needs met, and popular defense guaranteed. More than that, the PPLs were designed to involve the people in building their own revolution. While many people fled to refugee camps during the liberation of the region, many remained, hoping for some changes in their lives. This is how one FPL organizer explained the origins of the PPLs to me:

We found ourselves in territory in which there was the civilian population, the militias and the guerrillas. We realized that we had to deepen our revolutionary struggle and organize the population, to show them that, though the triumph hadn't come, nor had they lost the war. We had to find forms of organization which responded to the aspirations of the people to participate in the war. There was a vacuum in that sense; the people had been organized in the FTC,* but with the new situation, when most of the young people had joined the guerrillas, and others had joined the militia and everyone was talking about combat and military struggle, the masses were more or less stuck in the middle: "Well, and us, what do we do here? What is our role? Our role isn't just to go on *guindas.*"** They had come out of the political struggle which had first taken the form of economic demands for land, loans, markets for their produce; they had experience of an organization. But now they were in lands controlled by the people. From whom could they ask lands now or better salaries on the plantations? We had to respond to this new situation, to find a structure which would enable them to defend themselves from the

---

*The Federation of Rural Workers (FTC) was formed from the merging of the UTC and FECCAS in 1976.
**Guindas are mass withdrawals of the civilian population in the face of army invasions into guerrilla-controlled territory.

enemy offensives and to discover their own role in the revolutionary process.

For the peasants, the PPLs were the first chance they had ever had to run their own lives. There were five posts of responsibility in each PPL, plus a president and vice-president. Each post corresponded to a particular area of community life: social affairs (health, education), "legal" affairs, political education, defense, and production and popular economy. There were regular consultations with the villagers and each post was subject to frequent elections to give everyone maximum experience of administration. The intellectuals might return one day to run things, the peasants said, but at least they now had some experience to make sure their voice would be heard.

Inevitably, there were problems, and the success of the PPLs varied. A traditionally passive peasantry, with no experience of real democracy, does not gain confidence overnight. But there was no doubt that most of the peasants identified with their own form of local government. "How good it is to elect a president whom one knows personally," one peasant told me. "Not like before, when it was some unknown person who might turn up here, and we would know nothing about his life, his attitudes."

Metzi discusses some of the problems which arose in the civilian health programs, such as how to convince the peasants that there are other ways of dealing with health issues than with pills and modern medicines, traditionally denied them by poverty. But as Metzi makes clear, there are few easily available material or technical solutions to problems in the controlled zones; creativity is needed in all aspects of the revolutionary struggle. The tensions between the demands of the war and those of the revolution are present all the time. Militarily, the withdrawal of thousands of civilians during enemy invasions in the terrible *guindas* may not be sound practice. But politically, if the people are not defended, they will quickly lose faith in the revolutionary process.

By the end of 1983, the FMLN had the military initiative.

It controlled territory in about one-third of the country, in the north (Chalatenango, Guazapa, Morazán, Cuscatlán) and in the southern areas of San Vicente and Usulatán. The army could not maintain a permanent territorial defense in these areas, but limited itself to short-term incursions.

The bombing campaign which escalated at the beginning of 1984 was a response to the army's loss of the initiative on the ground. It badly affected the civilians living in the zones, the main victims of a tactic that the United States had urged on the Salvadorans in response to the inability of the army to defeat the guerrillas in armed combat. The bombings intensified during 1984 and 1985, at the same time as renewed efforts were made by the army to dislodge the guerrillas from their strongholds. Between May 1984 and the end of the year, the United States appropriated more than $260 million in military assistance for El Salvador, equivalent to the total amount of U.S. military aid to the country over the previous four years. The massacre of nearly fifty civilians at the confluence of the Sumpúl and Gualsinga rivers, which Metzi recounts in this book, took place during this renewed offensive.

At the beginning of 1985, Colonel Ochoa, a key figure in the extreme right of the Salvadoran Army, declared Chalatenango a "free-fire zone," telling reporters: "To help cut civilian contact with the rebels, the program in Chalatenango prohibits civilian movement or residence in twelve free-fire zones. Air strikes and artillery bombardments now are being carried out indiscriminately in these areas."* At the same time, a counterinsurgency civic-action program was launched in the department, with large amounts of U.S. AID funds for temporary job creation projects, health care schemes, emergency food aid, and relocation of displaced people. "It is the very same soldiers who after having burnt, destroyed, and broken everything which they have found in their way, are in charge of distributing food, clothes, and medicine to the people whom they have just hurt," a Salvadoran priest wrote to friends

---

**The Dallas Morning News*, January 21, 1985.

abroad about the civic-action programs in Chalatenango in 1985.

Low-intensity warfare and programs to win the "hearts and minds" of the population were now pursued with vigor nationally. In November 1985, the government announced its United to Reconstruct program, a government-controlled resettlement program in zones previously controlled by the FMLN. This onslaught, implemented by a much more sophisticated and professionalized army than that of 1981, thanks to U.S. training and equipment, succeeded in winning back control over some of the western part of Chalatenango. The army was now more willing to send smaller patrols behind the enemy lines and adopt more flexible counterinsurgency tactics, long advocated by the U.S. military advisers. In early 1984, U.S. pilots had begun flying surveillance flights over El Salvador at night, using laser detection equipment. This made it increasingly difficult for the guerrillas to move about in large numbers, although by that time they had brigades of hundreds of troops. The army now had very effective back-up from the air force. While in 1980 the country hardly boasted an air force, after 1984 it gained a fleet of sixty helicopters, thirteen A-37 fighter planes and five rapid fire AC-47 planes.

In January 1986, there were renewed army offensives against the civilian support base of the guerrillas in Chalatenango, Guazapa, and Morazán. Many civilians were forced to leave the controlled zones, particularly Chalatenango and the Guazapa volcano. The guerrilla struggle was entering a new phase. The guerrillas appeared to lose the military initiative, but Joaquín Villalobos of the ERP, probably the FMLN's foremost military strategist, has maintained that the shift in FMLN strategy was not defensive:

The next step for the FMLN was to move toward a more political strategy which would allow it to integrate political and military struggle. Here it is worth mentioning something very important: It was neither the air war nor the army's new mobile tactics which forced the FMLN to disperse its forces throughout the country. On the contrary, once it had broken through the army's defense of key centers, once it had built up military experience and leaders, and once a critical moment in the popular struggle had been reached, it would have been a very serious mistake for the FMLN to have continued waging the war only on its traditional war fronts, far from the people who live in the key urban centers.*

Militarily, the FMLN now organized its forces into smaller groups, operating over a much wider area of the country. This reduced the logistical problem, as it was much easier to supply a small guerrilla unit than a large brigade. Economic destabilization through acts of sabotage proved very successful, as Villalobos notes: "Our nation's small size, once seen as a disadvantage, now appears to be a great advantage for the FMLN. All strategic roads are within reach of its forces; as the FMLN consolidates and expands throughout the country and develops new forces, it gains access to all the roads nationwide. The same can be said about the government's electrical energy distribution system and the lands being farmed for export crops, which are the pillars holding up El Salvador's economy."** The FMLN began to reemphasize political work, particularly in the urban areas, rebuilding its clandestine networks in the capital. And occasionally it has carried out spectacular attacks to show it is still a force, such as the second destruction of the newly rebuilt El Paraíso barracks in March 1987, and the partial destruction of a major hydroelectric plant in May 1988.

Although the FMLN has lost territory, and no longer speaks in terms of "controlled zones" (a reduced area of eastern Chalatenango and Morazán north of the Torola river remain virtually under guerrilla control), in many areas, there is a situation of dual power. In some municipalities, the local administration collaborates with FMLN political organizations, sometimes with the knowledge of the authorities. In others, the FMLN has total control of the local administration, which can be disrupted by the army but not dislodged. In others, the officially elected local administrators can only

---

*J. Villalobos, "El Estado Actual de la Guerra y sus Perspectivas," in *Estudios Centroamericanos*, March 1986.
**Ibid.*

operate in the provincial capital, because the FMLN controls the municipalities. In this way, the FMLN still continues the experiment of the PPLs, although no longer under that name. In many local municipalities, the peasants are running their own communities in semi-clandestinity.

The failure of the United to Reconstruct program in the countryside to set up civil defense patrols among the population (as the Guatemalan army had done so successfully following its bloody counterinsurgency campaign of 1982) is largely a reflection of the high level of organization and political consciousness that exists, particularly in the north and east of the country. But it also reflects the failure of government reform plans, such as the agrarian reform, to make any real changes in the peasants' life. Occasional food handouts or temporary employment cannot substitute for a serious agrarian reform— one that provides the peasants with sufficient quality land and backs it up with credit facilities and technical assistance to enable them to feed themselves and their families. The dilemma for the Salvadoran government and the United States is that such a reform would have to start with a redistribution of resources away from the landed oligarchy and a reallocation of priorities towards the rural poor. Such action is politically unacceptable.

The most significant development in the last four years of the war has been the resurgence of the urban workers' movement and popular protest in the urban areas. A good deal of this has been spontaneous. According to the Economic Commission of Latin America, since 1983 real wages have fallen 55 percent among agricultural workers and 38 percent among other workers. Of every 100 urban workers of working age, only 27 have a fixed job and 80 percent of them earn less than the minimum wage. The misery of the urban poor has eroded support for the Christian Democrat government. The first strikes since 1980 took place in 1984 and 1985, and since then have become more frequent, better organized, and more militant. For the first time in many years, workers have taken to the streets to commemorate May Day and to protest government policies.

The earthquake of October 1986 deepened the urban crisis for the poor of San Salvador. It left 250,000 to 300,000 people homeless, most of them from the poorest sectors of the city. With the characteristic organizational capacity of the Salvadorans, many of the victims didn't wait for the inadequate government relief programs, but formed committees to fight for their rights. Many of the youth of the shanty towns are particularly combative. A new popular organization, The Bread, Work, and Freedom Movement (MPTL) is capturing their anger and militancy, as well as that of students and other urban groups, channelling it in ways reminiscent of, but not yet comparable to, the Popular Revolutionary Bloc of the 1970s.

In fact, the renewed combativity of the people is remarkable, given the context of human rights violations in which the popular movement has operated in El Salvador. Army massacres, death squad killings, and in recent years more selective assassinations have cost up to 60,000 lives since the war began. Yet despite the climate of terror and fear, the people continue to organize to defend their rights. In Morazán, whose recent history has been much less well documented than that of Chalatenango, peasant communities organized a peaceful demonstration of 500 people in 1987 and requested a permit from the 3rd batallion of the army to bring in food and medicines. The army believes their villages are guerrilla bases, but the peasants are asserting their right as civilians to live in their traditional homes. In the *"repoblaciones,"* the areas where displaced people have reorganized their communities under army vigilance, the population has similarly shown great courage in forcing the army to let food and building materials through.

While this activity of the popular movement is a response to the socio-economic reality in which the majority of people live, there is another story being played out on the political stage. The elections of March 1988 brought the far-right ARENA party to the center of that stage, giving them control of the legislature and signalling the demise of the U.S.-backed Christian Democratic project. They reflect the growing polarization in the country at large.

In El Salvador, the far right has a solid and quite consistent base of electoral support. But what is striking about the electoral contest of March is that only 35.7 percent of the potential electorate of 3 million (48.7 percent of the 2.2 million registered voters) actually bothered to vote. The electoral contest has ceased to have much meaning for the majority of El Salvador's population, particularly as the Christian Democrats have failed to bring either peace, reforms, or economic growth. The force that has taken advantage of this is the extreme right, which is likely to win the presidency in the 1989 elections. But the FMLN, which has always claimed that elections will solve nothing for the country's urban and rural poor, will also increase its following.

The FMLN still faces a formidable enemy in the Salvadoran army, backed by so much U.S. hardware. The threat of a U.S. invasion hangs over any thought of pressing for a military victory, even if the balance of forces were to shift decisively to the FMLN. However, the inability of the Reagan administration to send troops into Nicaragua suggests that in the post-Reagan era U.S. military intervention will be even less likely. For some years the FMLN has pressed for a negotiated solution to the conflict, but the government, confident of a military victory, has not taken negotiations seriously. Although President Duarte signed the Arias Plan, he has done little of real significance to implement its recommendations for a peaceful solution to the conflict. That plan did, through the regional political climate it created, enable some of the FMLN's political allies in the Democratic Revolutionary Front (FDR) to return to the country, opening up important channels of political communication with the middle and lower middle classes. However, the spaces which opened up during 1988 may be due as much to the confidence of the far right in its ability to control the situation in the country, as to any genuine liberalization or pressure for peaceful solutions to the civil war. Repression and death-squad activity escalated throughout 1988, and particularly since the victory of ARENA in the March elections.

The "people" factor in the Salvadoran war remains crucial to its outcome. The ability of the FMLN to present itself as a credible, viable, and acceptable political option to the impoverished majority of the population will determine its future. Militarily, the FMLN still has to make leaps from its situation of sabotage and harassment to one of almost continuous offensive, as was more the case during 1982 and 1983.

The guerrillas clearly have substantial support from the highly politicized and well-organized sectors of the peasantry and workers. This alone can explain the guerrillas' survival and growth over the last eight years. The renewed activity in the urban areas has helped the FMLN recapture some of its base there, though the space for the kind of political mobilization of the 1970s is limited, and a presidential victory by the extreme right ARENA party, with its history of association with the worst of the repression in the country, would limit them further.

More recently, the FMLN has begun to extend its activities to the west of the country, which since the failed and brutally suppressed 1932 uprising has been the least organized region and the one most susceptible to government manipulation. But many people in the area who supported the Christian Democrats in 1984 and 1985 are now disillusioned with the party and looking for alternative leadership. Given the objective conditions for the country's poor, it is undoubtedly possible for the FMLN to extend its base in these and other areas. But the power of the well-funded extreme right, with its clearly defined project of "pacification" backed by important elements of the armed forces and the private sector, should not be underestimated.

There can be no lasting peace in El Salvador until a solution is found to the problems of access to land and work, which led the peasantry and urban poor to take up arms in 1980. That solution will not be an easy one for whoever comes to power in the country, but if it does not involve the people and give priority to their needs and interests, war will continue. For now, the Salvadoran revolutionary movement remains one of the most significant of modern times; in reading Francisco Metzi's book, it will soon become apparent why.

Prologue

In late 1985, after having spent three years in the revolutionary-controlled zones of El Salvador, I went to look up some old friends. Traveling around Europe, Latin America, the United States, and Canada, I talked with a lot of people who were interested in the Salvadoran people's struggle. I was surprised to find that while I was full of optimism and sure of the liberation movement's possibilities of triumph, my friends were disheartened and badly affected by disinformation.

At first, I found this terribly shocking and couldn't understand their attitudes. But as I thought about it more, I began to ask myself: what had changed in me to separate us so? When I left for El Salvador, we had seen things eye to eye.

I soon began to realize that I had a considerable advantage: I had totally immersed myself in the everyday life of the men and women who are fighting a people's war. I had learned that "to love the people" was not just stereotypical leftist jargon. While these people taught me how to love them, I began to understand what a real revolution could be, and above all, I discovered day after day that the will to triumph exacts a very high price.

But the struggle itself had given me strength and vision. It rid me of a good part of the idealist conceptions that inevitably lead to disappointment and defeatism. Making a revolution was nothing like I had dreamed. The flesh and blood experience had made me see things in a new light.

My purpose is not to write the memoirs of an internationalist. As faithfully as possible, I have simply attempted to describe the immense difficulties and the exhilarating successes, the bitter disappointments and the real growth processes of this people to whom I owe so much.

My aim is that when you read in a FMLN-FDR communique about "our heroes and martyrs," you'll think of people like Freddy, Carlos, Juan, Lidia, and many others who are part of this testimony. When a wire service cable reports that "thirty-four civilians died during a vast army operation on suspected guerrilla hideouts," hopefully you will remember how we conserve our forces through strategic retreats that we call *guindas*. Furthermore, I've written so that you will more deeply understand the people's profound need for liberation through concrete images of life in communities like El Jocotillo, El Jicarito, and Tequeque, with their corn patches and their clinics.

I don't pretend to portray the Salvadoran people through images of extraordinary persons, but to show a collective struggle and the individuals engaged in it. I tell who we are and how we live in the midst of a people's war in El Salvador. My experiences provide the story line.

The war in El Salvador is fought on unequal grounds. We struggle to learn new skills while, at the same time, we scoff at the enemy's sophisticated technology. We began by using clubs for rifles and coconut milk for intravenous fluid. As we obtain medical supplies and requisition more weapons, we diminish the inequality. But even that would not be enough without creativity, sacrifice, on-going education, and above all, our will to win.

The people's war is a school for the society that emerges from it. Movement and change are continuous, not just in terms of geography, but also in form and structure. This book reflects firsthand experiences from 1983 through 1985; many of the problems described have since been overcome, or simply have changed. Such are the dynamics and the demands of the war.

The health struggle is prominent in my narrative since my work dealt with that area. I had relatively little training or experience in the field and so in this, too, the war was a school for me. I don't see medicine as a concern which is only of interest to professionals. Moreover, I understand health care as a window through which one can discover more concretely the multiple layers, old and new, of a society in the revolutionary-controlled zones, forming itself through numerous trials and errors.

Before going to El Salvador, I often reflected on what a revolutionary society could or should be; I asked myself about the relationship between justice and economic models, the role of the state, the contradictions between a strong party and grassroots participation. I was practically obsessed with keeping up on international events. In the war I didn't lose those interests, but the pressing need to resolve problems in the popular clinics, or the urgency of getting a seriously wounded patient out of the Front, was so strong that whole weeks would pass when I didn't even manage to listen to the news about our own struggle. My trench was the struggle for decent health care and in it I found my militancy.

That little something in all of us that is crazy drove me to a struggle and experience far different from the urbane lifestyle of the developed world that I had known. Now, as if that were not enough, I've undertaken writing a book in a language which is not my own. It was impossible for me to record my three years in El Salvador in any words other than those through which I experienced and internalized it. This has meant that Margarita, Flor, and Karla had to rack their brains not only to correct my Spanish and decipher my notes but often also to interpret them. As a result, the writing has suffered in terms of style, expressions and cohesiveness; nonetheless, I felt it worth the effort to feed back the story as I experienced it.

I hope that this book speaks to those who stand with the Salvadoran people, and that its testimony will strengthen their solidarity as it stimulates others to join in.

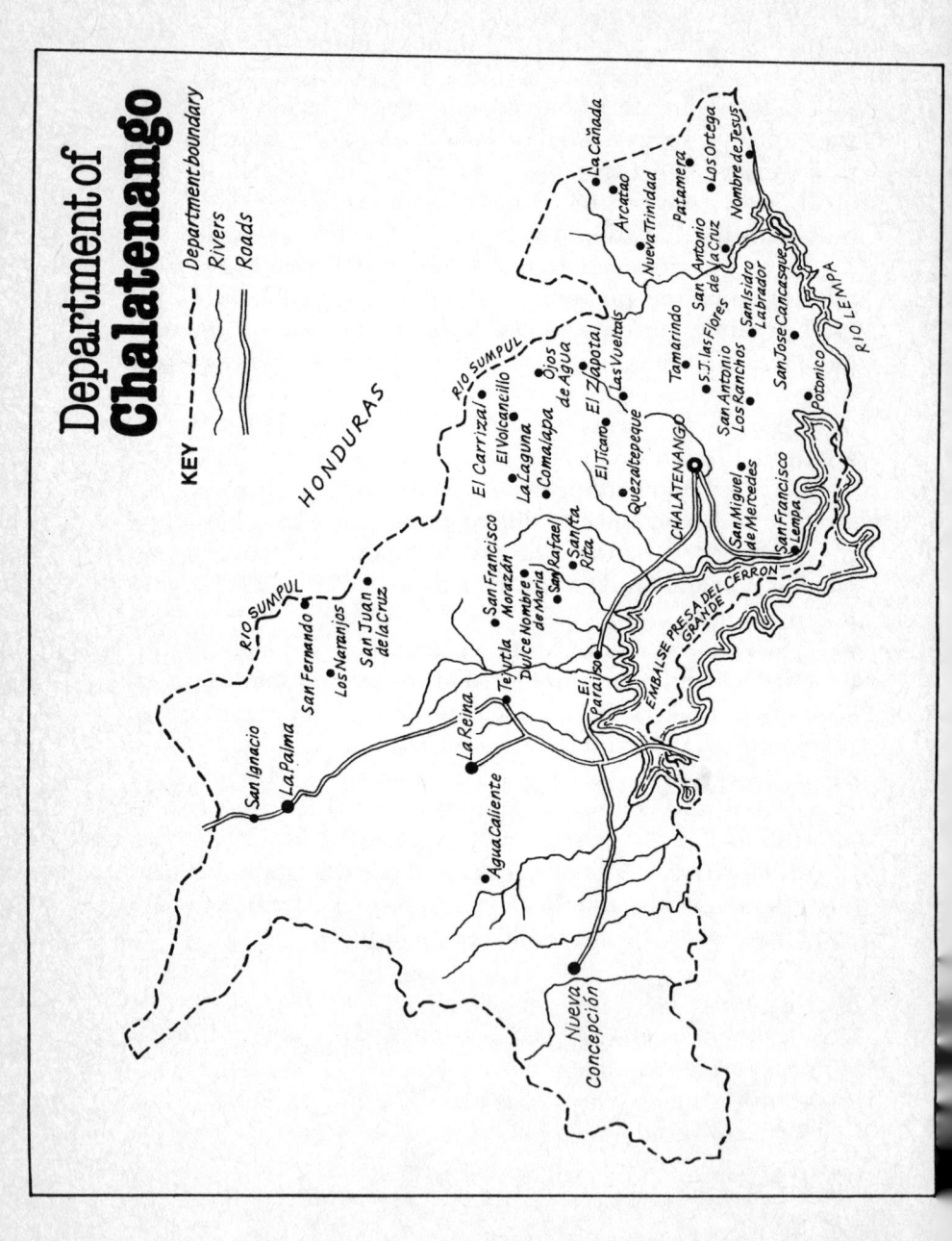

First Steps

I hadn't even been on the Front a week when Beto took me with him on his rounds as coordinator of three popular health clinics in the eastern part of the Sumpul Subregion of Chalatenango. We walked a good two hours to reach the first one, in Tequeque.

The clinic, more accurately described as a modest health station, was a small adobe house in the middle of a hamlet, where the villagers weren't armed guerrillas but undernourished peasants living in half burned-down or ramshackled houses. Instead of guns, they carried *cumas,* the typical short, rounded Salvadoran machetes.

Beto took great pride in showing me the clinic's medical instruments and supplies: the equipment consisted of a stethescope confiscated from an abandoned government health center, a blood pressure meter of dubious operational status, an enamel-coated bed pan, and several specula. Surprised by the specula, I asked if someone was doing gynecological checkups.

"No, *compa,*" Beto answered. "I retrieved these from the Health Center in Las Flores after the enemy retreated, but I don't know how to use them. Maybe you can teach me?"

I didn't have a clue how to use them either.

We then took a look at the pharmacy: a couple of small plastic bags with aspirin, an incomplete penicillin treatment, some pills for diarrhea, and a skimpy assortment of other pharmaceuticals. But it was clear that Beto considered four glass jars filled with red and brown pills to be the real treasure.

"What are these, Beto?"

"Vitamins and ferrous sulfate. We just got them. We've never had this kind of stuff before. They'll be the basis of a nutrition campaign we're organizing," he said, with great seriousness.

"Look, I don't know if you can run a whole campaign with just some pills," I dared to comment.

I was beginning to sense the immense gap between my ideas and the reality of a popularly-controlled health system.

"Well sure, man. Why not?" Beto replied with assurance. "Our people are underfed, right? And these pills are nutritional, aren't they?"

I tried to explain a few concepts about improving crops and food quality, but he interrupted me.

"How can we do that? We never know if we're going to harvest what we've planted. Understand? Look, I've got to get going and check up on the other clinic in Los Amates. It's a little out of the way and since you're not used to so much walking, why don't you stay here? You can orient the health workers, you know, explain a few things to them. I'll be back for supper and with some luck I'll bring some fish from the cooperative."

Beto left and I stayed with the two health workers, Elena and Yolanda. They decided to fix lunch before we talked. When it was ready, Elena handed me a plate with two tortillas and some bean soup, heavy on broth and light on beans. The two young women showed me to the table while they retreated to the kitchen doorway. I tried to get them to sit with me but had no more success than to provoke embarrassed giggles. I tried conversation, but that didn't work either. I think they felt as uncomfortable with me as I was beginning to feel with them.

After lunch, I suggested that we discuss their work. We sat at a table on the porch.

"What would you like to talk about?" I asked.

The two of them shyly covered their mouths and, lowering their eyes, stared at the ground.

"Perhaps there's some aspect of your work that's giving you problems. Maybe I can help?" I continued awkwardly.

They just blushed and had another attack of giggles. One more time. "There's nothing I can help you with?"

very uncomfortable. What's worse, they're a threat [to the] health of many patients, especially in cases of paraly[sis:] sores develop quickly despite the medical staff's watchful efforts. A hammock is much more comfortable; and, in the case of a lung injury, is actually better because it allows the patient to maintain a semi-upright position. However, a lot of the patients who might need resuscitation or those who had suffered a broken leg were obliged to spend their convalescence stretched out on one of these cots.

During a sadly long time, none of the *compas* in the ward managed to recover, so we dubbed them "The Regulars." Upon entering the ward, the first person you saw was Rafael, a big guy, just over twenty years old with long wavy hair that made him look like a hippie. But it soon dawned on me that there was nothing hippie about Rafael: he was pure Chalatenango peasant stock.

One day he told me that he didn't cut his hair because of a promise he had made. Once, when he was completely surrounded by the enemy, he vowed that if God helped him get out of the situation alive, he would never cut his hair. He was very serious as he spoke. But Juan and Medardo, both of them city boys and strongly influenced by Marxist thinking, would start in on him: "Cut that hair off, man! *You* got yourself out of that. You don't owe God anything!" But Rafael closed himself up in his beliefs and was faithful to his promise. Several years later, when he was among the disabled exchanged for President Duarte's daughter, who had been captured by the guerrillas, he cut his hair before leaving the country. What made him change his mind? I don't know. But what I do know is that in this war, slowly but surely, a lot of ideas get modified.

Rafael's brother, Mauricio, was well known all over the Front; a clever and willing *compa*, he was the head of the Los Amates Production Brigade, which includes a fishing cooperative, a dairy, vegetable gardens, and corn fields. Everything produced from these efforts was destined for the people's army, including the hospital. Through Mauricio we received watermelons, cucumbers, melons, tomatoes, and fish and milk for the wounded. This clearly gave Rafael a certain prestige among the other *compas*. Sometimes, when the goods came in from Los Amates, there might be a fish *pupusa*—a big tortilla pie which he was particularly fond of—just for him.

The others would tease him. "God, Rafael, it stinks of fish in here! Hurry up and eat that thing, man, the smell is killing us all . . . unless you want us to eat it for you." Then he would send it out to be heated up and share it with his neighbors.

But Rafael was not a cheerful patient. When the other *compas* would joke around with him, or when he would get something special, like the *pupusa*, he might brighten up a bit. But then, he didn't really have much to smile about. He had been shot in the upper part of the thigh, fracturing his femur. We had him in traction, using the primitive and ineffective system we had at the time.

The apparatus consisted of nothing more than a long narrow box for the leg to rest in, supposedly maintaining proper positioning. To create the required traction, we hung stones or bottles of water from the patient's foot. For what it was worth, the basic principles were there, but the results were lamentably poor. A more or less simple fracture could be set this way, yet since we didn't have access to x-rays, we had no way of checking the alignment. If the patient regained use of the injured limb, we would then consider it a "success."

With difficult cases, like Rafael's, the box system, which for some reason the *compas* had baptized "the helicopter," didn't do much. His injury was complicated when it became seriously infected. We spent several months trying to solve the problem, using up bottles of hydrogen peroxide and frightening amounts of different antibiotics. I remember giving Rafael, and other patients too, shot after shot of gentamycin with no result, making us wonder whether this batch was out of date, or if we weren't up against some super-resistant bacteria. We tried other drugs, but there still was no significant improvement. Daily we extracted puddles of foul-smelling pus from the wound; Rafael's thin blanket was almost always soaked and sticky despite regular washings. The thick bandages which we were obliged to use for lack of gauze, made from synthetic

Elena, the more daring of the two, finally said, "We just don't understand you."

"I thought there might be a few things that you were having difficulties with, and since I've had some professional experience. . . ." I talked slowly, making an effort to enunciate clearly. But this didn't get any positive results; on the contrary, it only provoked more nervous laughter.

"What kinds of diseases do you treat most?" I asked, taking a different approach.

But all they did was cover their mouths and shyly look around in any direction, as long as it wasn't in mine. I was upset, unsure of what to do next and feeling more and more like a foreigner, frustrated by the huge gulf between us. Somewhat desperate, I picked up a copy of the book *Where There Is No Doctor** and asked them:

"Have you read this book?"

Yolanda said something I didn't understand.

"What did you say?"

"I said, 'a little bit.' "

"Which parts have you read?"

"I don't know."

I opened the book to the chapter on intestinal parasites, repeating my question, but I still couldn't get a direct answer. I kept on, paging through different chapters, but that was not an effective way of establishing communication either. What's more, I was beginning to realize that Yolanda was just barely literate and Elena couldn't read at all.

"How is it that you became health workers?"

They looked at each other to see who was going to respond. Without even lowering her hand from in front of her mouth, Elena answered, "Beto gave us a course."

"What did he teach you? What topics did you cover?"

"What what's?"

"Topics. What did you talk about?"

Elena thought for a moment. Once again she consulted Yolanda with a glance.

---

*David Werner, *Where There Is No Doctor* (Palo Alto: The Hesperian Foundation, 1977).

"You know, about medicine . . . everything. Curing wounds, diarrhea, fevers, flu, malaria, coughs, infections. That's all."

"How long was it? The course, I mean."

"Five days."

"Five days? That's all?"

Elena didn't understand my surprise. "I mean, that's a lot. We had to go all the way to Patamera every day, you know." Patamera was another hamlet, a good two hours' walk away, made difficult by steep, rocky slopes.

"Why didn't you just stay the night there?"

"Well, our families wouldn't let us. Besides, you never know when there'll be a *guinda*.* It's dangerous to be far away."

"And the people here need attention," added Yolanda.

"Why don't we have a look at the pharmacy?" I suggested.

"If you say so."

I picked up a bag of sulfonamides. "What are these used for?"

"For diarrhea," responded Elena.

"Nothing else?"

"Well, no."

"Okay, these are good for some kinds of diarrhea; but, can't they be used for other things like urinary tract infections, for example?"

They looked at one another, as if to ask, "what is this guy up to?" Elena felt encouraged.

"Well no, not exactly. For an infection you use penicillin. Now for this ur. . . uri. . . . What is it?"

"Urinary tract infections. Like cystitis, for example. When it burns when you pee."

"Oh, you mean 'burning piss'! For that we use Bactrim."

"Yes, you can use Bactrim. It belongs to the same family of sulfonamides."

"No, I don't think so. I mean . . . sure, well, if you say so."

I started to lecture on sulfonamides and antibiotics: what they're used for, how you can substitute one kind for another if

---

Guinda is the popular word used for a strategic retreat undertaken by civilians and the revolutionary forces in the face of an invasion by governmental troops.

The Insomniacs' Collective

There's just one thing our hospitals in the revolutionary-controlled zones have in common with those in developed countries: the name. Ours are not spotless silent towers of science. You won't find long corridors where people huddle together, sharing their sorrow, nor orthodox wards submitted to the TV's authoritarian stare, nor white curtains separating patients from one another's suffering.

A guerrilla hospital is more like a neighborhood café, where friends get together after a late night political meeting to discuss the results of the latest ball game. It's a lively place, even if you bear in mind its share of pain and sorrow.

The atmosphere of the hospital varies with the rotation of patients and their personalities. During the three years that I spent in the war, one of the most memorable periods was at the hospital near Tequeque.

This medical station was located in a typical adobe house. Some of the wounded and non-critically ill patients slept in hammocks on the porch. Since it was "summer"—the dry season—the slightly wounded patients and the staff would sleep on the ground, either in the patio or on the earthen floor of the house. The heart of the hospital, however, was the ward—a twelve by twenty-four foot room, where the most difficult cases received attention. Here the patients slept on *tapexcos*, cots made from bamboo poles slit lengthwise and roped together with vines, which are then placed on a fixed frame planted in the ground.

Sleeping on one of these improvised beds is a challenge even for the soundest sleeper. The surface is totally uneven and you have to. Soon I noticed that Yolanda was staring off into space, not paying attention at all.

"Aren't you interested in this, Yolanda?"

"Oh, yeah, sure," she said, and they both started giggling again. I continued my lecture. A few moments later, Yolanda leaned over and whispered something to Elena.

Feeling a growing confusion, I stopped talking. It was apparent that these girls had a lot to learn, yet they didn't seem to show the slightest interest.

"Are you following me?"

"What?" Giggles.

"You know. What I'm teaching you here, is it interesting?"

"Oh yeah, yeah, sure," responded Elena evasively. Then suddenly she asked, "Is it true that in your country it gets really cold and snows?"

I felt utterly incompetent to do this kind of work, and something deep inside me told me that I had better ask to be sent to work in the hospital as quickly as possible. There I would be able to do whatever they assigned me while I gained some time to figure all this out. There things wouldn't depend so much on my own initiative, as was the case with teaching; and in a hospital I wouldn't feel so useless.

We all got up from the table. The two young women went about preparing the fire to cook sorghum* for the tortillas. I went inside to lie down for a few minutes. From there, I heard Yolanda say, "I hope Beto brings fish because we don't even have any beans left to offer him."

---

*Before the war, sorghum was cultivated mainly as fodder for domestic animals. Only the poorest peasants used it for human consumption, once their corn crop was depleted. Now, with the war, it is the cereal from which tortillas are most commonly made; its nutritive and culinary value is inferior to that of corn.

very uncomfortable. What's worse, they're a threat to the health of many patients, especially in cases of paralysis. Bedsores develop quickly despite the medical staff's watchful efforts. A hammock is much more comfortable; and, in the case of a lung injury, is actually better because it allows the patient to maintain a semi-upright position. However, a lot of the patients who might need resuscitation or those who had suffered a broken leg were obliged to spend their convalescence stretched out on one of these cots.

During a sadly long time, none of the *compas* in the ward managed to recover, so we dubbed them "The Regulars." Upon entering the ward, the first person you saw was Rafael, a big guy, just over twenty years old with long wavy hair that made him look like a hippie. But it soon dawned on me that there was nothing hippie about Rafael: he was pure Chalatenango peasant stock.

One day he told me that he didn't cut his hair because of a promise he had made. Once, when he was completely surrounded by the enemy, he vowed that if God helped him get out of the situation alive, he would never cut his hair. He was very serious as he spoke. But Juan and Medardo, both of them city boys and strongly influenced by Marxist thinking, would start in on him: "Cut that hair off, man! *You* got yourself out of that. You don't owe God anything!" But Rafael closed himself up in his beliefs and was faithful to his promise. Several years later, when he was among the disabled exchanged for President Duarte's daughter, who had been captured by the guerrillas, he cut his hair before leaving the country. What made him change his mind? I don't know. But what I do know is that in this war, slowly but surely, a lot of ideas get modified.

Rafael's brother, Mauricio, was well known all over the Front; a clever and willing *compa*, he was the head of the Los Amates Production Brigade, which includes a fishing cooperative, a dairy, vegetable gardens, and corn fields. Everything produced from these efforts was destined for the people's army, including the hospital. Through Mauricio we received watermelons, cucumbers, melons, tomatoes, and fish and milk for the wounded. This clearly gave Rafael a certain prestige among the other *compas*. Sometimes, when the goods came in from Los Amates, there might be a fish *pupusa*—a big tortilla pie which he was particularly fond of—just for him.

The others would tease him. "God, Rafael, it stinks of fish in here! Hurry up and eat that thing, man, the smell is killing us all . . . unless you want us to eat it for you." Then he would send it out to be heated up and share it with his neighbors.

But Rafael was not a cheerful patient. When the other *compas* would joke around with him, or when he would get something special, like the *pupusa*, he might brighten up a bit. But then, he didn't really have much to smile about. He had been shot in the upper part of the thigh, fracturing his femur. We had him in traction, using the primitive and ineffective system we had at the time.

The apparatus consisted of nothing more than a long narrow box for the leg to rest in, supposedly maintaining proper positioning. To create the required traction, we hung stones or bottles of water from the patient's foot. For what it was worth, the basic principles were there, but the results were lamentably poor. A more or less simple fracture could be set this way, yet since we didn't have access to x-rays, we had no way of checking the alignment. If the patient regained use of the injured limb, we would then consider it a "success."

With difficult cases, like Rafael's, the box system, which for some reason the *compas* had baptized "the helicopter," didn't do much. His injury was complicated when it became seriously infected. We spent several months trying to solve the problem, using up bottles of hydrogen peroxide and frightening amounts of different antibiotics. I remember giving Rafael, and other patients too, shot after shot of gentamycin with no result, making us wonder whether this batch was out of date, or if we weren't up against some super-resistant bacteria. We tried other drugs, but there still was no significant improvement. Daily we extracted puddles of foul-smelling pus from the wound; Rafael's thin blanket was almost always soaked and sticky despite regular washings. The thick bandages which we were obliged to use for lack of gauze, made from synthetic fabrics found in abandoned villages, were inadequate because they were nonabsorbent.

So on entering the ward, the first thing that hit you was the terrific stench. But no one ever mentioned it in front of Rafael. Only he would make sick jokes about how the worms were going to have a lot less work when he died.

Once, a new lay nurse removed the bandages for the daily treatment, and as the awful smell invaded the room, she cried out in the most spontaneous and insensitive tone, "Oh my God! Does that stink!" The entire ward wanted to belt her, and though no one made the slightest comment right then, they didn't easily let her forget her crack.

"Do I stink too?" they would tease her when she came around to change their bandages.

We were faced with a really serious problem: we needed an orthopedic specialist. Since no antibiotic seemed capable of halting the infection, we presumed that it was caused by a sequestrum, the medical term for a piece of dead bone trapped between healthy parts. Without x-rays and without knowing what kind of bacteria were present, no one dared operate.

I don't know exactly how the problem was finally resolved, since I had already left the hospital before Rafael was well enough to go home. One day though, I met him on a path; I was thrilled and, at the same time, surprised to see him so far from his village.

"Look! I'm back in business," he exclaimed.

He then stood up straight, like a soldier at attention, and barked "ten-shun!" In that position, you could see that the wounded leg was some three inches shorter than the other and completely deformed. I stared at his leg for a second and then the two of us started howling with laughter, hugging and slapping each other on the back with a really bizarre sense of joy.

Neto had the *tapexco* next to Rafael's. He was a combatant with what had originally appeared to be a minor wound in the leg, but in the course of tending it, we discovered that a large vein had been damaged. He too had to spend months and months on his back waiting for his leg to heal. Sometimes the vein would start to bleed spontaneously, and he'd go into shock. We would bitch and swear in the poorly illuminated ward while trying to perform the most basic procedures: apply a tourniquet, start him on an IV, and monitor his vital signs.

Like the other *compas*, Neto liked to help pass the long, idle hours listening to music. I had some cassettes with songs by Violeta Parra, Daniel Viglietti, and Carlos and Luis Enrique Mejía Godoy which, when there were enough batteries, we would listen to in the dark. These were especially moving times for us. Even though they had never heard Violeta Parra's music before, the *compas* immediately adopted it as their own. On the other hand, they were already familiar with a few of Viglietti's songs. "*Pedro Rojas*," based on César Vallejo's poem about a combatant who fell in the Spanish Civil War, was such a success that it left everyone silent, pensive, and very moved. The Mejía Godoy brothers' "*Guitarra Armada*" generated enthusiasm and comments. Radio Venceremos and Radio Farabundo Martí, the guerrilla radio stations, played it frequently, and everybody loved it. We would then discuss Nicaragua with familiarity and tenderness. We talked about how they had won the war, about their struggle against the *contras*, about their internal contradictions. I think we all felt a certain envy toward Nicaragua, free Nicaragua. Those songs evoked the insurrection, and with them they brought back memories of the huge demonstrations in San Salvador in the 1970s; spontaneously our confidence in our future triumph would come pouring out.

Neto had developed a remarkable memory, perhaps as a consequence of being barely literate. Just by listening to a cassette once, he'd have a couple of the songs memorized. The second time, he'd perfect his first try and start on several more. He spent hours on his bamboo cot, a thick hemp rope suspending his leg from a roof beam, reciting lyrics half out loud, and later singing them softly. As time went on, we hardly needed the tape player; day or night, Neto would nourish our lives and our dreams with the songs recorded in his mind, while waiting for his war-shattered leg to heal.

On a nearby cot lay Medardo, a twenty-two year old ex-student who had been in his first year at the university when he joined the guerrillas in San Vicente. He had come to Chalatenango in 1981 as part of a select group of combatants chosen to form the very first Vanguard Units.*

He was wounded at Miramundo, a mountain near La Palma in the western part of Chalatenango, during a battle which had been led by a U.S. advisor. With the bullets whizzing all around them, our radio operators intercepted a message from enemy headquarters, giving the order to withdraw "that hick." "Which hick?" responded the enemy field radio. "The gringo, you son of a bitch!"

Medardo had wounds all over his body, but an open fracture of the tibia was what was causing all the problems. It had become seriously infected, resisting all treatment, probably also the result of a sequestrum. In spite of all our attention and treatment, only time eventually closed it up.

Contrary to most, Medardo was extremely self-critical about having been wounded. At Miramundo he had ordered his platoon to retreat when the fighting got too heavy. But as his troops fell back, they abandoned a real gem, a 90mm recoilless cannon which not only had been confiscated from the enemy, but was one of the very few we had. He had instructed a squad to go back and retrieve it, but they refused to follow his orders and challenged him to do it himself. Our troops are very demanding and insist that an officer be willing to follow through with any of his own orders.

In view of the situation, Medardo crawled back in pursuit of the weapon while the *compas* covered him with their fire. Despite being exposed to the enemy's guns the whole way, he recuperated the cannon and was dragging it back when, just a few short yards from safety, he was hit by grenade fragments.

I didn't understand why he was so self-critical; it seemed to me that his wounds were unquestionably honorable.

"Of course, you can't understand; this is all just an adventure to you."

"What the fuck is this adventure shit, man?"

---

*The Vanguard Units are the most qualified units in the people's army.

"Well, just that, you, you don't think about what it means to build an army. But we do. We think about it a lot and heroism doesn't interest us. I should've been able to make those guys follow my orders."

At night, Medardo, Juan, another wounded combatant, and I would argue for hours on end, sometimes raising our voices to a brotherly aggressive pitch. We would talk about many things: our personal views on life, the revolution, and the war. Ours was a confrontation between Europe and Central America, between the loosely-organized, anti-authoritarian activist and the Marxist-Leninist guerrilla. But these were important moments in getting to know each other, and it was, above all for me, the perfect chance to get closer to these people, their struggle, and the concepts behind it.

Once I asked Medardo what he wanted to do after we had won. He didn't hesitate in responding. "Keep killing Yankees, continue the struggle against imperialism. That's how much I hate it for what it's done to our people."

No one spoke. Medardo's words and steady voice filled the darkness. "We have to kill. It's an essential part of the struggle. But even though imperialism forces us to do it, we mustn't get used to it. There should always be some weird feeling, something ugly about killing."

He was fascinated by books, an indiscriminate reader who believed that the theme didn't matter, any book deserved to be read in one sitting. Later he would discuss what he had read with the others.

Once, while reading aloud a passage about the struggle in Guatemala, one of the other *compas* turned on the radio. Medardo stopped reading and stared at him. "You won't solve your own problems or win the war by listening to pop music," he said, picking up the reading where he had left off. Without a word, the *compa* turned off the radio.

Another time, when I was feeling down and lost, he called me over and said, "Look, pal, when we've won this business, and the country is free, me and my buddy are going to take you to every single nook and cranny of the coast and then you'll see that it was really worth it. How about it?"

Unfortunately, Medardo won't be taking me around free El Salvador. He later died, victim of a piece of shrapnel that lodged in his heart when he was hit during an air raid attack.

Medardo's neighbor and the last in that line of bamboo cots was Juan. He was an internationalist whose right leg had been amputated. "One-legged Juan," as he was called to distinguish him from the others, had been wounded during an attack on La Laguna, a fairly important town on the road to Chalatenango. He had only been on the Front for a few months when he took part in the assault on the National Guard post there. Hugging the walls of the neighboring houses, he was able to get right up to the command center and plant a charge that blew open the back of the building. The *compas* were then able to go in and take all the guardsmen prisoner. But as he withdrew, a bullet hit him in the leg.

The wound itself was fairly run-of-the-mill, not even a fracture. But the following week, our territories were invaded by 18,000 Salvadoran and Honduran troops—the famous *guinda* of November 1982, a very difficult period indeed. God only knows why, but within a few days Juan's leg became infected with gangrene. This dreaded infection was pretty rare on the Front; in my three years, I only saw two cases.

It was a period in which we were very short on medical supplies. We didn't even have IV fluid. Under these conditions, an amputation is a delicate operation, and even more so in the presence of a ferocious germ. But in spite of all this, we operated on Juan under a silk-cotton tree, cutting through the bone with the tiny sawblade of a Swiss Army knife, and using the milk from several coconuts as IV fluid.

Juan became a "regular," not because of the amputation but because of a rare skin disease that developed first on his extremities and then little by little took over his whole body, including his face. It would clear up in one spot, break out in another, and then spread back again. Even today, we still don't know what caused it. However, it was finally decided that, cured or not, Juan should leave the hospital and be assigned a new task. Slowly, after he had been working for a few months, the infection disappeared and only recurred insignificantly from time to time over the following years.

Juan loved life and had always been very active, full of energy. It must have been a tremendous effort to adapt to the amputation, but he never mentioned it. He spent long hours just sitting quietly and I imagine that during those moments he was forming a new image of himself.

I remember once, during a meeting when the patients were strongly criticizing the lay nurses, Juan spoke up, "Look, maybe I'm one-legged because somebody made a mistake, or maybe that has nothing to do with it. I got all caught up in that for a while and I felt bitter. But, later, I said to myself: Fuck it! What difference does it make now whether someone screwed up or not? We're at war and war is a series of some steps forward and others backward. The important thing is to win. And, no matter how it has to be, even as amputees, or as fucking basket cases, we can keep this process moving if we put our minds to it."

After leaving the hospital, he was assigned the delicate task of controlling logistics routes, a desk job which he joked about, calling himself a "guerrilla bureaucrat." But as an active revolutionary, just twenty-five years old, who wouldn't have trouble getting used to being such a "bureaucrat," vulnerable to any invasion? Whenever there was an enemy offensive, he had to be moved to the rear guard on horseback. That worried me. What would happen to him when that wasn't possible? I'm sure everyone was asking the same question, including Juan. But he never brought it up. With affection, and out of consciousness and love for life and the struggle, Juan not only accepted losing his leg, but did so where mobility was a strategic necessity.

There was a fierce invasion in September 1984 on the day on which some of our wounded were to be sent abroad for treatment in exchange for the release of captured enemy army officials. We were forced to hide our wounded, including Juan, in a cave. Sitting out an enemy offensive inside a shelter is about the worst thing that can happen to you in a war: not only is it extremely uncomfortable, but you feel like a sitting duck.

Juan had been given the chance to be included in that exchange and leave the country, but he rejected the offer; he wanted to stay in what he felt was the right place for him. But in the next invasion he wouldn't hear of going to another cave; he and his security squad went and hid in an out of the way spot, thick with bushes and brambles.

On the last day of that invasion, an enemy patrol began combing the area. There was no way an amputee could get out of there alive. Juan argued bitterly with the *compas*, forcing them to leave him behind. With the enemy closing in, he attempted to retreat, but his crutches broke once he entered the bushes. He only had a 22-caliber pistol and two grenades; one of them didn't explode, the other did.

After the invasion was over, we found what remained of him about 600 feet from where the security squad had left him; his skull simply didn't exist any more, nor did his hands. His chest was riddled with bullets. It seems that the soldiers had called for him to surrender, "You're not going to get anywhere with that water pistol."

Like so many others, Juan had understood that "Revolution or Death" was not just a slogan. Aware of the strategic information logged in his memory, how could he possibly allow himself to be taken alive?

While in our "Regulars" ward, Melvin had the cot opposite Juan. His story exemplified another element of the drama we lived in the people's war. He was a militiaman from Veragua, the brother-in-law of Morena, the village health worker. They were both devout Christians who had joined the popular forces precisely because they had understood the communal message of Christianity. They had met Archbishop Romero when he'd visited their village, and had worked with Ita Ford, one of the four nuns murdered by a right-wing death squad in 1980. Their commitment to the revolutionary movement was strengthened, among other reasons, when they saw how such exemplary people were simply gunned down in cold blood.

One night, as Melvin was getting up for guard duty, his large caliber, pre-World War I rifle fell and accidentally went off. The bullet passed through his right thigh, injuring an important vein. Morena applied a tourniquet and managed to stop the bleeding. But during all the months he spent in the hospital, the vein repeatedly and spontaneously hemorrhaged massively. At any moment of the day or night, a member of the staff could be seen hurrying to answer Melvin's pathetic cries for the tourniquet; it finally got to the point where we just left one there permanently, ready for any emergency.

Changing Melvin's dressings was always a challenge. His anxiety made him tense and totally obsessed with his wound. He complained about everything, and if, during the treatments, the slightest touch made him wince, he would jerk our hands away. More than once I had to holler at him just to do a routine check.

But the *compa's* condition was serious. As a result of the repeated hemorrhaging and the largely insufficient diet, he had become severely anemic. At that time a transfusion was out of the question, and to make matters worse, maintaining aseptic conditions was very difficult. The wound was soon badly infected. The bullet's trajectory had now become a veritable cave. At least three times the granulation tissue managed to reach the skin surface, but each time the goddamn vein would burst again, and, of course, the infection would set in once more, setting us right back to zero.

Things got progressively worse. Melvin's blood pressure went up to 180, either as a result of his anxiety or as a perverse reaction to the constant hemorrhaging. At the least provocation, even when he just tried to make himself comfortable in his cot, the bleeding would start all over again. Often a bowel movement was enough to bring on the hemorrhaging. Since privacy as such didn't exist, there was no alternative but to relieve yourself right there in front of the other patients, lay nurses, visitors, and whoever else might happen to be there at the time. Being extremely shy, Melvin would wait until dark to take care of his personal necessities; but his prudishness was frequently frustrated, since the necessary effort often provoked the bleeding, which in turn resulted in a terrific scandal, waking up the whole ward.

The other *compas* would tease him with their black humor. "Tonight, Melvin, we want to get some sleep. We forbid you to take a shit!"

Embarrassed as well as fearing another attack, Melvin would constantly restrain himself. So we'd have to order him to defecate. "Do it two or three times a day, but for the love of God, Melvin, don't get constipated!"

He lost hope of ever getting better and thought he was going to die. Our diagnosis was not all that pessimistic; yet, in view of the limitations, we couldn't offer him any real hope, either.

When Melvin's desperation became dramatic, the other *compas* tried to encourage him with their own special solidarity, a mixture of realism and black humor.

"You're gonna die, Melvin, you're gonna die!"

I remember being horrified by this scene when Melvin suddenly began speaking as he never had before.

"All of you are here because you were doing something worthwhile. You were wounded in battles for our liberation. Me, I'm here wasting medicines that should be going to combatants, taking up this space and the doctors' time because of my own stupidity!"

Juan answered him with irony. "Kick him out of here! Get his butt out of the hospital! This guy is taking up a combatant's place. He's a civilian and they don't do anything except feed us!"

Medardo chimed in. "Shit, man! What the hell are you talking about? You know we're all in this struggle together. We're all fighting for our liberation, all in our own way, civilians and guerrillas alike. Don't you feel scared shitless sometimes when you're on guard duty? Isn't it as courageous a way as any to defend your people?"

This shocking conversation turned out to be amazingly therapeutic. Melvin had isolated himself in his depression and feelings of inferiority. After this incident, he was more self-confident; he felt like he was one of the *compas*, too.

He eventually did get better. We were able to get enough medicine to stabilize his blood pressure, and the vein finally healed. He was one of the happiest patients I ever saw leave the hospital.

"What luck! I still have enough time to prepare the corn field. My family won't go hungry on my account."

Another of the regulars was Napo. He was a metallurgist and had been assigned to the armory and logistics. After a successful attack, he had been driving a captured truck full of confiscated weapons when the vehicle became the target of the first rocket blast in a sudden retaliatory air raid. Napo and Andrés, the *compa* riding with him, were seriously burned. They only survived because the explosion catapulted them right out of the truck.

Andrés was in shock and unconscious when they brought him in. He had third degree burns on his arms, face, torso, and most of his legs. It was impossible to find a vein to give him an IV. We finally succeeded in dissecting into a vein, using the tube from a butterfly-needle infusion set as a makeshift catheter. Under normal conditions, a patient like this is isolated in a strictly sterile environment. We put him in the most "antiseptic" place we had: the operating room, despite the risk of contaminating it. But this was one of those hopelessly painful cases where there is nothing else to do but wait for death.

A pseudomonas infection set in, with its horrible color and characteristic odor; he got worse and worse, until his breathing indicated that he was in a state of complete electrolyte imbalance. He was in such misery, we were relieved when he died.

The suffering of his companion was different. Although Napo had burns on his face and all over his arms, most of them weren't third degree. His face wasn't even that bad, but flies somehow managed to lay eggs on his forehead and in the corner of one of his eyes, next to the tear duct. When he started complaining about something "biting" him, we examined him closely and discovered the first maggots.

Although it wasn't common, the medical staff always took it very badly whenever a wound got infected by maggots. On the one hand, it is positively anguishing to see those creatures squirming in a patient's flesh, and to be obliged to cause him even more suffering by plucking them out. On the other hand, we considered it our fault that the flies were able get at the wound.

To kill the maggots, we usually resorted to the same poison that the local peasants used on their livestock. But in Napo's case this was out of the question: for one thing, we didn't have any, and even if we had, it would have been too risky applying it so close to the eye. In such cases, we relied on an extract derived from fresh ground basil, which wouldn't kill the maggots outright but would cause them to surface. The green liquid causes the insects slowly to emerge; at that instant, you have to pluck them out one by one with a tweezers. However, it isn't as easy as it sounds, since the tail end of a maggot forms a screw that allows it to keep a strong grasp on the flesh. If you don't snatch it firmly the first time, it will bury itself, hiding deep inside the wound again. It usually takes eight days to get rid of them all. Only once the infested part had healed could we really be sure of our success.

Due to the poor lighting inside the hospital, we had to carry Napo outside for these sessions. An infested wound attracts flies like fresh dung; so our team had to include a lay nurse whose sole job was to wave a rag around, keeping the flies at bay.

After treatment, Napo spent the rest of his day in his *tapexco*, unable even to sleep from the pain and the discomfort. His face was completely bandaged, making it difficult for him to communicate with the others. But the *compas* took it upon themselves to make sure that he had cigarettes, "anaesthesia" as they called them, especially during the daily cleansing. There was something almost comical about watching him puff on cigarettes through a tiny slit in the bandages, the smoke coming out somewhere around where his nose was buried under the layers of gauze. "Maybe I can suffocate the little bastards," he liked to joke.

What most concerned us was that the maggots might attack the eyeball itself. But we were lucky; within a week we had won the battle, and within a few more weeks Napo was back at his job.

Many other *compas* had to idle away weeks or whole

months stretched out on their bamboo cots: multiple fractures, chest or abdominal wounds, appendicitis, typhoid, you name it. But others were able to convalesce on the porch or in the patio and would wander through the ward, chatting with the patients and the health team. A few of these were "Regulars" as well, including Emiliano, who had been hit by a bullet from a G-3, a large caliber West German rifle, destroying his cheek and lower jaw. Not only was this a terribly painful wound, having affected the trigeminal nerve, but it also meant that he couldn't eat solid food, which he found humiliating.

His best buddy was Pablo, "The Cat," whose minor flesh wound in the thigh became infected, postponing his departure from the hospital.

Irremedial insomnia is common among the wounded, but these two crazy characters used it as an excuse to party all night long. At any hour of the night, you would find one or the other wide awake telling wild stories, talking about girlfriends or buddies, or teasing other patients. They loved to josh the lay nurses and doctors. One of their most memorable exploits was a "Patients' Union" they organized, complete with officers whom they would choose and remove at whim. The main function of the Union was to guarantee the patients a steady diet of watermelons from Los Amates, when and in the quantities they established—and not as Julia, the head of the hospital, programmed. Late at night you could hear them chanting the Union slogan: "What do we want? *Watermelon!* When do we want it? *Now!* "

They called their insomniacs' collective "The Big Sleep." They could smoke a whole carton of cigarettes in a single night, despite the doctors' warnings that smoking would slow down their recovery. The Union had its own private channels for obtaining cigarettes and would oversee their distribution.

"The Café" was another one of the Union's schemes during this period. Because there was always the possibility that more wounded would arrive at our already too small hospital, Julia, a nineteen-year-old peasant woman with three years' experience as a guerrilla lay nurse, decided to expand the unit. Behind the patient's ward there was a tiny porch which housed the adobe oven used to sterilize the medical instruments. The idea was to create a space where a few more bamboo cots could be set up, by extending the tile roof and walling it in with straw fixed onto wooden frames.

Why this project was never completed, no one really knows. Little by little, however, the more mobile wounded used it as a place to hang their hammocks, seeking out the shade there in the heat of the day. It was Medardo's and Juan's "study," where they would read whatever they could get their hands on, while sipping the coffee brought by their special "contacts." Before long, "The Café" became the perfect spot for endless discussions among the patients, staff, and visitors: topics varied from the Allende years in Chile to policies of China and the Soviet Union; the viability of armed struggle in Europe; the development of imperialism and Salvadoran history; and included every imaginable theory about when and how we would march into Plaza Libertad in San Salvador to celebrate our triumph. Sometimes the discussions heated up and we would take to calling each other reformists or revisionists or some other Marxist "insult." And, occasionally, someone with real expertise would hold a mini-seminar.

But we didn't just talk politics; we all took turns narrating our favorite movie, relating an anecdote, or confessing our "most embarrassing moment," which usually brought on the laughter, comments, and criticism of the others. We didn't think of it as anything solemn or serious; more than anything else, it was just another chance to cultivate the affection that exists among comrades.

It was a café without beer or booze; the only "illegal substances" we had were those that Juan and Medardo got from their contacts: coffee and cigarettes. The Union meetings were a way of making life as bearable as possible for both the wounded and the hospital staff. In the midst of the weariness and hopelessness, without worrying about all the danger and suffering waiting for us out there, we made life itself one hell of a party.

One Day They Asked Me If I Wanted to Be a Guerrilla

Injured in 1983, Emiliano left the Front some months later so that more expert hands in better hospitals could finish treating the damage done to his jaw and cheek. In this interview, he gives us his peasant's point of view on being wounded and contributes to our knowledge of the incipient guerrilla movement in 1978–1981.

Where were you wounded, Emiliano?
It was during the attack on Tejutla. Some *compas* had laid an ambush along a dirt road, and I was part of the back-up troops. About eight o'clock in the morning they radioed that the enemy had fallen into the trap and ordered us to start closing in from behind. But when we got up there, I saw nothing but soldiers coming down on us. I was yelling instructions to another *compa* when I felt a jolt. It didn't hurt at all, I just sensed a blackness coming over me. "Well now," I said to myself, "isn't death just fine?," and I lay there unable to move. A little while later, the feeling came back in my hands and feet. "I'm OK," I thought.

"We're gonna get you out of here," a *compa* cried to me.

"No. If you guys try and get me out, you'll get yourselves killed. Keep me covered, I'll get out of here on my own."

I got up all right, but I had lost a lot of blood and didn't even make it thirty feet before I began to faint. I saw a *compa* without a gun so I gave him mine; this wasn't so unusual since it was still during the time when there weren't enough weapons to go around. I managed to go a little further but I fainted again, landing practically at Medardo's feet.

"Jesus, they really fucked you up, man!"

"Yeah, I guess so."

"Well, that's war for you. Before you know it you're dead."

"Ain't that the truth. This time I think I've completed my mission."

I hadn't even gotten the words out of my mouth when the enemy soldiers surrendered. There were fifteen of them. The fucker who had hit me came over and tapped me on the shoulder.

"Sorry about the bullet, man."

"Don't worry about it," I told him through my teeth, but I really wanted to finish him off. I was so pissed because now that he had surrendered, I couldn't kill him.

The pain didn't really get to me until we reached the medical station, and then, shit, man, it was the worst! Jose was in charge there.

"You're bleeding pretty badly. There's about five blood vessels that need stitching. I'm going to try to fix that, so just remember, it's for your own good."

He stitched two but I couldn't take it and started kicking and giving him hell until he finally laid off. When I'd calmed down a bit, he came back. But as he was finishing, I started in on him again. It's like that, you just can't control yourself. Later, when I was a little more myself, I apologized to him.

"I'm used to it. All you guys give us hell," he answered.

A little later, one of the women brought me a soft drink from Tejutla. I tried to gulp it down, but it just ran right out the gaping hole in my cheek. I could taste it, but nothing was going down. "That's some hole," I thought. "This thing's never going to close up." That night when I checked it out with my hand, I felt so badly I started to cry.

Finally, they took me to a base camp where they did a "horse-doctor" cleaning on me.

"This might hurt," Mario, the doctor in charge, told me. "Just hang in there."

Two women had to hold me down while they scrubbed my face with a surgical brush until it bled. I kept my eyes closed so I couldn't see what they were doing.

They didn't use any anaesthesia?

No, there wasn't any. Not until three days later when we got to El Común did they give me a shot of local anaesthesia.

The wound was really foul. Since the only way I could sleep was on my back, I ended up swallowing a lot of pus. I asked Mario if this was bad for me. But since he was always clowning around, he responded, "No, man, you're on antibiotics, it won't hurt you. In fact, it's probably good for you."

The trip to the hospital in El Tamarindo took two whole days and while we were on the road, the *compas* carrying me fell and I rolled down a hill.* Man, that was so fucking painful! When we got to a town everybody bought sweet rolls, and, shit, man, they even fried some eggs! Mario bought me a soda to dunk the roll in, but I couldn't even open my mouth. My lips were huge and my tongue was swollen right up against my palate. Not only that, I was beginning to have trouble breathing. You could say I was in pretty bad shape.

Even in the hospital, at first it was nothing but liquids. Later I graduated to puréed beans, but no tortillas. Not eating tortillas is like not eating at all! My jaw was nothing but broken pieces that the doctors were unable to put together. With the slightest movement I got this horrible rush of pain.

I remember once when I was on call you asked me for something for the pain. All we had was aspirin. I felt so badly and remember thinking, "What the hell are two aspirin going to do for him?" But you didn't complain.

It helped; it would ease the pain for a little while. Later, when we finally got some injectable painkiller, I decided to drink the shit right out of the vial, since my arms already hurt so much from all the penicillin shots. God, was that stuff awful! After that you gave me drops. I would start to sweat, feel real groggy, and then, hey, I felt just fine.

---

*Injured and severely ill patients are transported by means of a hammock slung on a bamboo pole and carried by two persons, one at each end, the pole resting on their shoulders.

And you kept asking for more! The medical team was worried that you would get addicted. How did you feel when you saw your face?

I measured the hole everyday with one of my fingers until it finally got down to the size of my little finger. I checked it out in the mirror, too. I still wanted to be a combatant.

When I left the hospital the wound itself had finally healed, but my jawbone had been so badly destroyed that the doctors were unable to set the fracture. Even though it didn't hurt anymore, it still hindered my talking well and eating with ease.

But things didn't get real hard for me until I went back to my battalion. Two days after I got there, the others all went off on a mission and left me behind. I told the officer in charge that I wanted to go with them, but he said no, I needed to rest. I just sat there all by myself and cried that whole afternoon. That night I dreamed I was fighting, but when I woke up I was alone and could hear the machine guns off in the distance. "Shit," I thought, "maybe I'm no good anymore." And I started getting real neurotic about it. Later on, I told one of the platoon chiefs that I thought they were fucking me over. He then talked to the ranking officer and that same afternoon he brought me a gun.

"Look, you're coming with us. But you're not going to the front line. You're gonna stay back with me so you can give me a hand if necessary."

That was great, just what I needed to get over my crisis.

You come from a peasant background, right? What made you join the struggle?

It was in 1978 in San Vicente. All around people were joining up. Before that, I didn't know anything about the guerrillas. I had heard some talk about guys with guns and stuff, but I didn't know what they were fighting for. I hadn't even been involved with the grassroots organizations.

One day a cousin of mine came over and just plain asked if I wanted to be a guerrilla, to carry a gun and fight. I said, "Sure!" so he took me to a meeting where they asked me if I was willing to fight to liberate my country. "And what's that all about?" I asked them. They then explained what revolution meant: change the country, get rid of the system that we have now, and make one where everyone would participate and say what he wanted. That's more or less what they told me. I got the picture, so I said OK; it sounded good to me.

These were guerrillas?

No, they were militiamen. There was a bunch of them, but they didn't have any weapons—not one. They would go out with a stick in a burlap bag making it look like a gun. They would attack the "rats"—local reactionary spies—with these "weapons" and then turn over the real ones they confiscated to the guerrillas. Or they would hold up rich folks in their cars on the highways, charging them a toll. Just think of it, stopping the cars and humiliating the people, making them think that those were real guns. That's how it all started.

Almost as soon as I got to the San Vicente volcano I started to realize what the hell it meant to fight. In three days we only ate twice. There was an invasion and we had to make a run for it right up to the very top of the volcano. As new recruits, we were armed with nothing but clubs. In the whole platoon, there were only three hunting rifles, two 22-caliber pistols, and not much else except plain old machetes.

What kinds of actions were you doing at that time?

We were keeping the area clean of "rats," and we confiscated food and clothing for civilians and the guerrillas. One time we went to one of the big ranches looking for this "rat" who was working for ORDEN.* The guy's son was a *Guardia*, but supposedly he never showed up at the house. We got there just around midnight, knocked on the door, and suddenly realized that the house was crawling with *Guardia*. They started firing at us and we didn't have any guns. The officer in charge ordered me and another *compa* to position ourselves alongside one of the windows. Bullets were flying all over the place and I was scared shitless, standing there with only a machete. "We're not going to last long this way," I said to myself. I was beginning to learn just how hard the struggle was.

Pretty soon, one of the *Guardia* started firing a submachine

---

*The Spanish acronym for the Democratic Nationalist Organization, an extreme-right rural paramilitary organization.

gun out the window. In just one chop with my machete, I left his hand dangling there. I grabbed the machine gun, and saw the guy trying to get away. Since I didn't know how to load the thing, I chased him with the machete. When I caught up with him I gave it to him in the back. He wasn't going anywhere now! Then I turned the gun over to the officer, who was the only one among us who knew how to use it.

So that's how it was with just about all of them that night. We confiscated clothing, weapons, even a tape recorder, and we left a leaflet vindicating our action. That night we must have finished off about eight of them. It was the first time for me, and I felt something really ugly about killing like that.

How did you justify that action?

Their job was to check up on the workers. If they suspected you of collaborating with the guerrillas, they'd kill you without batting an eye.

Was the BPR* organizing on that farm?

Yeah, the majority of the people were organized in the BPR and had complained about the foreman. After we cleaned up there that night, the organization talked the new foreman into improving conditions and salaries. He agreed because if he hadn't gone along with it we would have burned down the farm. People began to gain confidence in us and we were able to broaden our base of support.

What would you do with the civilians when the governmental army invaded?

Once, during an invasion, a bunch of civilians came right into the base camp asking where to go and what to do; the army was all over the place. We told them that if we all hung together, and were real quiet, we could break through the cordon and get out by Playa Piedra, but it would mean walking all day and night.

There were about 400 people in all. We assigned security guards to the front and rear. At one point, we came real close to running right into the enemy. They were just on the other side

---

*The Popular Revolutionary Bloc, which united a vast number of trade unions and other grassroots organizations.

of a stone wall, talking and fucking around. We all crouched down and no one made a peep for a long time, until they finally moved on. Some of the folks wanted to get closer and see how many there were, but the head guy kept making signs for everyone to stay put.

A little later, we reached a big ranch, where the enemy really got us. They were deployed on two hills on either side, with us in a riverbed right in the middle. Everyone hit the ground and started to crawl, even the pregnant women. Everytime a grenade exploded, another baby was born. (Laughing.) You know, the shock and the fright! The women just got the baby out, wrapped it up, and kept on running. In the end, we managed to get away under the cover of some corn fields without a single casualty. The next morning we finally got to Playa Piedra. That's how the people gained confidence in us; they saw that we wouldn't just run off and leave them.

Did you take part in the January 10, 1981 offensive?

Of course. They told us this was it—victory! Everyone was real gung-ho. I got some good training, special forces stuff, and they gave me one of the only M-30 machine guns we had; it had been requisitioned from the enemy just a few weeks before. I was part of the attack on a big town, Zacatecoluca.

When the time came, I didn't even take any clean clothes, thinking I would change after we had taken the town. In a nearby village, Siete Joyas, we joined up with a lot of other people, civilians who were armed only with sticks with a nail in one end. The people were really excited, everyone believed this would be the victory. There were about 150 of us; some were to stay behind as back-up, the others would attack the army post, and the rest, the National Guard base. I was in that group. The first truck made it through the road block all right, but they nailed us and started firing. I couldn't even figure out how to get off the truck with the machine gun. I was scared shitless. I finally just threw myself off, firing like a madman.

Some of the civilians threw homemade fire bombs, so that the flames would cover us from the enemy as we crossed the streets. We worked together like that for a while but when the enemy opened fire on them, they had to get out of there. stayed on in town but since our experience wasn't in urb fighting, a lot of *compas* ran off and hid in houses. I ended up alone with the platoon chief, and before long a tank came down on us. The thing was only about thirty feet away, but I was so petrified I couldn't even fire. I didn't take cover or anything, I just stood there.

What made you do that?

I didn't give a fuck whether I died or not. Bullets were flying all around me.

The platoon chief shouted at me, "Show 'em you've got balls, man! Keep shooting."

"Fuck, man, I'm not scared; that's why I'm standing here like this," I told him.

Finally the chief fired a G-3 rifle grenade at the tank, and we watched it go up in smoke. Right about then he got hit, and I had to fight hard to get him out of there. We made it to a house, but instead of opening the door, they started shooting at us. I thought there must be soldiers inside. "Fuck this shit!" I said and kicked in the door. Two more shots, and then, Christ! It was a bunch of *compas* who had taken cover there. Among them were some lay nurses. I was really pissed and started screaming about how this was a real war, and they had to do something for the chief. I took over and we spent the night there. There were soldiers on every street corner.

How did you get out of there?

We borrowed a dress from the lady who owned the house and I sent one of the *compas* out to the Red Cross to get a car; her story was that her husband had been wounded by a stray bullet.

When the ambulance got there, I told the Red Cross worker that we were guerrillas and we had to get out of there.

"The Red Cross doesn't take anyone who's armed."

"Right, but now it does. We've got to get this guy out of here. In the public hospital they'll kill him."

We loaded the *compa* in the ambulance and took off, honking and waving white flags out of both sides. We went right through six roadblocks. As soon as we were out of town we stopped. I thanked the driver. "Don't mention it," he said, and we took off into the hills.

That night we found a house where they gave us some food. We explained that we were guerrillas. "That's great," they said, "we've been helping you guys. If you want, you can stay here tonight." But we had to get back to the base camp.

When we did get back, the head of the Front came up to me.

"Shit, man! I thought we had lost that M-30."

"Over my dead body!" I answered him.

Was the other attack more successful than yours?

Yeah, they were able to get into the base. They didn't take it over, but the people were better organized. The next day they attacked the power station.

How did you feel when you realized that the offensive had failed? What did the people say?

Most of us were pretty disheartened, but the *compas* said that it was a good experience. "We confronted the enemy, and even though they were much better armed than us, we almost won. We can't let this get us down," they said. Some people did desert. Many civilians were pretty disillusioned. They became very cautious about supporting us. We had pushed them too hard. But later, when they saw that we were still out there, they gave us their support again, and we got their confidence back.

War is like that, you know, you win some battles and you lose some. But in the end we will bring this enemy to its knees.

Our Own Hospital

Hospitals in the controlled zones play an important role for the civilian population, as well as for the people's army and the party. In this sense, they are real institutions in the life of the whole Front.

When a hamlet is chosen as the site for a hospital, it gains a certain prestige and soon becomes a center of collective life. When the hospital moves, the villagers feel disappointed and sad. They often continue to keep up the house where it was located, in hope of its return.

Once, in Tequeque, while scouting for a location to hold a seminar, a *compa* told me, "There's always the hospital. It's still vacant, just in case you decide to come back."

Before the war, the rural population had to travel to hospitals in the cities to receive medical care. Nowadays, living near one of ours guarantees medical attention, but at the same time constitutes a risk, since hospitals are prime enemy targets. Even so, the people always speak proudly of "our own hospital."

Everyone has contributed something towards its construction. The civilians have pointed out the safest location for it and then helped build it. They have also helped carry the wounded there; the crops from their fields have supplied its provisions. As for the militiamen and the combatants, they have risked their lives to protect it, while teams from logistics have lugged heavy backpacks full of medical supplies over dangerous backwoods trails. In this respect, the hospitals are the result of a community effort, a symbol of the people's accomplishment.

But, as the war went on, we felt the need to have clandestine hospitals. This proved to be truly difficult in such a small and densely populated area as El Salvador. It is impossible to set up a new facility without at least a handful of local people knowing its whereabouts.

Once, in a supposedly secret hospital, we were resting just after having finished abdominal surgery on a combatant, when a group of locals brought in a woman in a hammock.

"We know we shouldn't come here, but the *compa* is really sick. So we decided to risk it."

The patient turned out to be a thirty-year-old civilian with acute appendicitis. There was just one thing to do: put ourselves into high gear, wash and sterilize the instruments, and prep her for the operation. It was 11 P.M. before we finished. If the people had waited, if they hadn't considered the underground hospital their own, the woman's appendix would have ruptured, probably killing her.

On any given day at the hospital, one could see civilians and *compas* from the different workshops, recovering from an operation, a bad bout of malaria, or a battle with typhoid. I can't even recall how many caesareans we had to perform.

However, it was primarily in the outpatient clinic that the relationship with the civilian population really took shape. Working there played an important role in my personal development. It was there that I learned to diagnose and treat common complaints; and even more importantly, I got to know the people in the midst of their liberation struggle.

As many as twenty-five people came in a single afternoon. The consultation wasn't limited to discussing the patients' ailments; it often included whole chapters of their life stories and family problems as well.

By January 1983, most of Chalatenango was under revolutionary control. As a result, those who had fled during the nightmare of government repression overcame their fear, left the refugee camps, and went back to their fields and homes; the lucky ones found their houses still standing. During all of 1983 and the first half of 1984, the civilian population grew until it had quadrupled.

Those who had been in refugee camps managed to recover somewhat from a life of chronic undernourishment and were not quite as unhealthy as those who had remained behind, holding out despite the war. The ex-refugees usually consulted us for specific complaints, such as an infection in the digestive, respiratory, or urinary tracts, for all kinds of parasites, or for different sorts of rashes or fungal infections. By contrast, those who had stayed showed up looking pale and yellowish from anemia, aggravated by constant bouts of malaria. Their hair had long since lost any semblance of shine, and they looked like walking skeletons. The children were underdeveloped for their ages, their bellies swollen from worms. Although there were some cases of acute malnutrition, most just suffered from prolonged undernourishment, which never reached a critical stage.

These people had learned to get by on whatever they could find in the hills. Only on rare occasions had they managed to supplement that with the basic foodstuffs common to the rural population: beans, corn, and more often than not, sorghum. Even if they had money, they couldn't run the risk of going into one of the villages to buy supplies. Their diet had consisted of roots and leaves, unripened fruits, the pulp of banana and papaya tree trunks, and any wild animals they were able to hunt.

Upon examining them, we found chronic diarrhea and undernourishment, parasites of every class and color, and a wide variety of aches and pains. Any hope of laboratory analysis was pure fantasy; our only basis for diagnosis was clinical observation. Taking medical histories was very complicated, since few had precise recall of past illnesses and the popular rural vernacular they used to describe their ailments was incomprehensible to us city-bred professionals.

The only real advice we could offer most of the patients was to try to eat better. "I'll try, *compa*," they would respond with incredible patience. To save the situation from being too absurd, I attempted to give them some encouragement, "That's one more reason to win this war."

"We've made a lot of progress. It won't be long now," was the inevitable response, born of a confidence that was really hard to understand at first, considering everything these people had already been through. "And anyway, we've got the corn planted and they aren't taking it from us this time!"

One of the complaints I most often heard was, "I get out of breath easily on the slopes." The terrible truth of that phrase didn't hit me until I, too, was anemic and understood the flesh and blood challenge of the hills.

Chalatenango peasants can walk for hours over rugged terrain without tiring, and at a pace that can wear out even the best-fed, best-trained European. As I had watched them carry fifty pound sacks or wounded *compas* up and down the backwoods trails, I felt admiration for this underfed people. It reaffirmed my belief in their capacity to resist and defeat their enemy, right down to the last Yankee. So when they did feel worn out, that was reason enough to seek out a doctor.

Often, in order to make the long trek from an outlying village to the hospital, people would band together in small groups for safety's sake. On one occasion, a big group from several of the hamlets to the south arrived, laden with presents for the patients: honey, fruit, *tamales*, coffee beans, and corn. What extravagance! These items were not just scarce, most of them were virtually priceless. Everyone was overjoyed and we prepared a little ceremony to welcome the visitors and express our thanks.

When it was over, Carolina, one of the doctors, asked me if I would give her a hand, since, surely, most of them would want to make the most of the trip by seeing a doctor. Within a few hours, sixty people had passed through our hands.

Unlike doctor's office visits elsewhere, there were none of the usual appropriate facilities for making examinations and so, unless the exam was of an extremely intimate nature, it was done in public. Everyone could hear the doctor's advice given to the other patients, and they could take advantage of these conversations, using whatever was pertinent for themselves.

Especially in front of strangers, Salvadoran peasants are very modest about their bodies. The way they overcame this bashfulness was admirable. For example, diagnosing diarrhea meant asking a lot of embarrassing questions: "When you go to take a shit, do you fart much? Are they really stinky?"

This direct way of doing things soon became the rule. Intimacy gave way to a collective lifestyle, as an essential condition for survival.

Parties were another important link between the community and the hospital. Many occasions were an excuse for dancing; this passion, even in the war, has not been lost in El Salvador.

The best parties around were the ones at the hospital, probably because so many young women worked there. Male *compas* from all over the subregion would show up just to dance with them: from the explosives workshop, the military training school, the information and propaganda office, and the Subregional Government Council. It wasn't surprising to see some guerrilla commander taking a few hours off to dance with the lay nurses, and then, just like most of the others, walk several hours back home to be at work the next morning. The rest slept at the hospital; on those nights, doing rounds meant navigating around piles of bodies sleeping directly on the earthen floor in the ward and all down the porch.

There was a dance during the time of the "Insomniacs' Collective" at Tequeque which made a big impact on me. That afternoon a young boy, the son of one of the *compas* in charge of the PPL, the local popular committee, had been critically wounded in the leg. He had stepped on one of our own land mines while out picking mangos beyond the security parameter.

We amputated his leg in a futile attempt to save his life, but he died on the operating table. Not just the medical team, but everyone at the hospital felt sad and defeated, even though we hardly knew the boy.

Suddenly Emiliano grabbed a guitar and shouted: "No crying! Come on, everybody! Let's dance!"

Right there we started dancing, as if for our lives, a frenzied dance as vital as the liberation struggle itself. And while we danced with such passion, Margarito kept watch over his dead son, the third he had lost to this war. We didn't leave him alone; the people would go in to view the body, accompany him for a while, and then go back out to join the dancing.

Somehow there was always music for the parties. Usually

Arturo or Emiliano would sing and play the guitar, but even if we only played the same old cassettes using some worn-out batteries, nothing would stop us from dancing. There were also a couple of musical groups in the controlled zones. The biggest and most well known was from El Sicahuite and boasted two or three guitars, a bass, two violins, and Don Ramiro, the poet-singer of the group. Another band, "*Los Farabundos*," were a real folksy, lively group that knew exactly how to please the crowds.

Bandaged eyes, heads, arms, or legs didn't stop the *compas* from dancing. I even remember watching amputees dance, one arm holding a crutch and the other around a partner, while they both roared with laughter. And since a guerrilla fighter never puts down his or her gun, the image of these couples slow-dancing in each other arms was as tender as it was bizarre.

When we danced to the music of these bands, we shook to the rhythm of the progress of our guerrilla forces; far from causing us to forget our political perspective, these parties strengthened it. From the middle of the dance floor, we periodically shouted revolutionary slogans, reflecting how our commitment permeated all aspects of our lives.

These interludes also gave us a chance to improvise little theater pieces about the major events in the country. Someone mimicking Reagan would call Duarte on the carpet for having bungled the defense of the big hydroelectric plant, Cerrón Grande; then in the next scene, there would be somebody playing Vides Casanova, the Minister of Defense, or Blandón, the Military Chief of Staff, getting a tongue lashing from Duarte. Sometimes, in a party given the last day of a workshop, we used this theater dynamic to summarize the contents of a seminar. Certain elements of these pieces, such as composition and props, actually contained principles of avant-garde theater.

At one memorable party, two guitarists from Tequeque livened things up by playing local country music with their own revolutionary lyrics. But after a while the tone changed; the Union began insisting that Julia, the head of the hospital, sing one particular song. At first, she refused to acquiesce, even though normally, without too much pressure at all, she would sing for hours on end.

Finally, she started singing in a strong passionate voice, but in no way would she satisfy their special request. In the end, one of the wounded took the initiative and began to sing it. To the immense joy of all the patients, by the second verse, Julia had joined in.

I didn't understand what really had been going on until much later: the song was a play on words with a none-too-subtle reference to the female sex organ, and Julia had quite a reputation for her amorous tangles. Despite the crudeness and machismo, I was impressed by the people's frank vitality. Even in the most ordinary circumstances, the desire to live life to the fullest has made the Salvadorans a strong and struggling people.

The Lessons of El Jocotillo

I had heard about Paulo Freire for nearly a decade but hadn't ever taken the time to read any of his work. After all, I was not a teacher.

In fact, I was as ill-prepared to understand social phenomena as I was to teach or even to give medical care. I knew something about medicine and had gained a little experience working in a hospital, which led me to believe I could be an asset to the revolutionary movement. However, that proved terribly presumptuous on my part. In order to be truly useful to the people of El Salvador, I first had to learn from them, and only then did I begin to contribute to their struggle. A workshop that I gave to local health workers in El Jocotillo served as a giant step toward understanding this.

I was quite lucky; just as the seminar began I got my hands on a copy of *The Pedagogy of the Oppressed*. For the first time I found myself participating as an educator and learner among the oppressed who, in this case, were primarily young women from the surrounding poor agricultural communities.

I was impressed by Freire's writing, which corresponded to a lot of my own feelings about life and political struggle; however, I couldn't find anything practical that would help in my new job as a teacher. The idea of "problematizing reality" sounded great, but how was I supposed to do that with the large intestine, or symptoms of malaria? How was I going to engage in dialogue about tapeworms and the proper medication to treat them?

My first impulse was to dismiss Freire's ideas as inadequate in our context. This left me with only traditional teaching methods, which turned out to be increasingly unsatisfactory. What else was there to do? I began to doubt that I could teach these young women anything. I found myself ruing the day I got myself into this war, so high on dreams and so low on the stuff that makes them come true.

In the middle of class one day, it suddenly occurred to me that I was looking at the problem completely backwards. It wasn't these young women who should sit back and absorb what I taught, but rather, I should learn from them. After all, these women were local experts who had suffered all their lives from the very diseases that we were studying. This "discovery" radically changed not only my teaching style, but also my relationship to the community as a whole.

I began to see the human body and health care the way the peasants understood them; this proved to be the key to making my work more useful.

For example, we were talking about diarrhea one day when one of the young health workers asked me if I believed in the "evil eye." How could I? I didn't even know what it was.

So I learned that, according to popular beliefs, children don't die as a result of dehydration caused by severe diarrhea, but rather from a spell cast by the "evil eye." Any number of people possess this dubious power, particularly those with physical deformities such as a withered arm, a blind eye, or a hunchback. Pregnant women can also acquire it.

The curse manifests itself in a severe case of diarrhea, accompanied by a high fever; usually, the child dies within a few hours or days, unless the "spell can be broken." All the health workers gave examples of relatives and neighbors whose children had died in this way.

The cure for the "evil eye" depends on magic, too. The most common remedy is to rub the child down with rue, or swab its body with sweat wrung from the father's, or some other special person's, workshirt. This person must be chosen with great care, otherwise the spell will worsen. People also believed that if the mother puts the child down while she goes about making tortillas, death can move in and take advantage of this negligence. Not all the health workers agreed on the remedies for the "evil eye"; several didn't believe in the curse itself. Those who doubted it the most were precisely the ones who had been most influenced by the new ideas that the war had fostered.

To me these old wives tales seemed repressive, guilt-provoking, and at the same time, dangerous, particularly given the fatal effects of diarrhea. Nonetheless, they provided me with some strategic information for introducing new ideas and proposing a more adequate plan for treating diarrhea.

The peasants believed that their illnesses were due to prolonged exposure to the sun and to the heavy rains that they were forced to endure, especially during *guindas*. Once I had to cut short a visit to another hamlet because the militiaman who had accompanied me insisted repeatedly that we head back early so as not to get drenched in the habitual afternoon shower. He had been treated for gonorrhea and despite my explanations, he continued to attribute it to a soaking he received during a retreat.

For the most part, any illness was interpreted as a punishment for not having respected an established norm. Rheumatism, bronchitis, and many skin diseases were explained as the result of "taking a bath before my body had cooled."

There also was a strict code of behavior. If she doesn't follow the prescribed rules, a pregnant woman can miscarry or bear a deformed child, and a nursing mother's milk will dry up.

Becoming familiar with these beliefs proved invaluable to being able to treat the population. Medical science holds that frequent bathing is the best way to avoid fungus infection. Yet, it was no use advising a *compa* with ringworm to bathe when he came in from the fields in order to wash off the sweat and soil. He wouldn't do it. However, if I suggested that he take a quick bucket bath, soaping up only once to ensure that he didn't get chilled, I might be successful.

A lot of the ideas about sickness and health seem to have been inherited directly from Hippocrates and European medical knowledge, as introduced by the Spanish Conquerers. Heat and cold are the most important elements, or "humors," although air plays a basic role as well. "I'm certain I was attacked by an 'air,' " explains muscle aches and rheumatism for many. Remedies are classified according to which "humor" is involved in the ailment.

Consequently, amoebic dysentery with only mucus must be treated differently than when mucus and blood are present. Mucus is "cold" and blood is "hot." If I recommended lemon, which is "cold," as a remedy for both, I was screwing up in the eyes of the locals. Even so, not everyone agreed on the hot or cold nature of different ailments or on their respective cures.

Enlightened by discussions held in the workshop, I was able to learn the different names people used for their common complaints and to help the health workers identify parasites by using their own symptoms as a basis for classification, while I came to realize that real symptoms were not always mentioned in the medical texts at hand.

This teaching method which I had "discovered" had its political importance, too. In a war where the poor start from scratch and slowly plant the seeds of their own liberation, gaining self-confidence is imperative. All the combatants agree that this is a crucial step.

In health care the process is identical. Starting from the base of knowledge that already exists among the people, even if it is not always interpreted correctly, contributes to building that assurance. Lack of self-confidence was most often expressed in the form of shyness. "I don't know anything. We don't know . . . you're the one who knows, you should tell us": this attitude was antithetical to my teaching approach. Political and military leaders frequently exhorted all of us to conquer this shame since it was an expression of oppression within ourselves. In the fight to overcome it, Elizabeth and Morena, two health workers with above average political consciousness, became my allies.

Perhaps the most difficult obstacle of all was the peasants' blind faith in industrialized medicine, in pills, and "even better, an injection."

Raquel, a forty-year-old widow, tried to convince me that her failing memory was due to a lack of vitamins. That might have been true at one time, but over the course of three years, whenever we saw each other she came up with the same request for vitamin pills. In this respect, Raquel was a true reflection of popular theories: vitamins are "nourishment," and since the people know they are undernourished, they buy them to improve their health. The domestic pharmaceutical companies specialize in tonics and vitamin supplements, proclaiming their virtues in frequent radio and newspaper advertisements.

Arnulfo, the shoemaker, was a good example of the consequences of this: he complained of constant headaches, soreness, and general exhaustion. I attributed it to an inadequate diet, perhaps to a lack of B vitamins. But his aching increased, and when he began talking about fevers and pain in the small of his back, I feared he might have a kidney infection, which prompted me to prescribe Bactrim before it could get worse. I gave him the medication at about four in the afternoon.

By noon the next day, a changed man stood before me. "Paco," he said, "you gave me a miracle drug!" It wasn't just his health that had improved, but his whole attitude, and all in less than twenty-four hours!

Arnulfo's miraculous transformation was due to his unshakable faith in pills, compounded by the fact that I prescribed drugs that he knew were in short supply and thereby had confirmed his own importance to the war effort.

The strangest case I saw in El Jocotillo was Lisa, the militia chief's wife. I went to visit her when one of the health workers told me about her rheumatism, which was so severe that she couldn't get up for days on end.

She was fortyish and lived with her husband and daughter in a small house just off the path. She greeted me effusively, explaining that she had been suffering from this affliction for years and just couldn't stand the pain anymore. She couldn't sleep at night, and her complaining kept everyone else up too. She assured me that the pills the health worker had given her made her feel better, but not nearly so good as those that she had once received from an army medic. She showed me a sample that she had carefully saved and assured me that, with just one in the morning and another in the evening, her pain had been alleviated. I was perplexed. Lisa had been taking ampicillin which, in that dosage, couldn't possibly have had any real effect on chronic rheumatism.

When I discussed the case with the health worker, she told me that Lisa was notorious for her attempts to get pills from anyone, saving them up and taking them according to her own self-prescribed schedule. I also learned that although she hadn't dared to expose her bad temper to me, she frequently gave the health workers hell, threatening them until they gave her medicine.

Lisa was indeed a neurotic and tyrannical depressive, who used her condition to manipulate people. I tried to change her relationship both to her illness and medication, but it was an utter failure and all ended in heated discussions. As a result, soon after, she forced her meek husband to use his position to organize a hammock team to carry her to the hospital. But my reports had prepared them for her arrival; she was given a placebo treatment and in a few days, she was up and around, feeling fine. Regrettably, the last I heard, nearly two and a half years later, was that she had once again sent her husband to the main pharmacy to secure pills, entrusting him with another precious sample, this time, of prednisone.

Self-medication is common throughout the country: it allows people to avoid having to pay a doctor's fee or wait in line at a health center. One can purchase pills and injections without a prescription in just about any store. Drugs are even hawked by vendors on intercity buses. How much one buys depends on his or her pocketbook, and self-diagnosis determines the variety. "Don't you have any pills for malaria or for a cough?" was the inevitable question people asked doctors and health workers alike. Of course, a few cough drops can't cure a congested bronchitis or tuberculosis.

Not all the patients were like Arnulfo and Lisa; most of them were victims of deficient diet. After the government offensive of November 1982, the Front as a whole, and particularly the area in and around El Jocotillo, was left in a catastrophic condition. The whole population was forced to flee, abandoning practically the entire bean crop still out drying in the sun. The enemy doused it with gasoline and set it on fire.

The almost ripe sorghum fields were also destroyed. As a result, foodstuffs could only be obtained in the less devastated areas. This obliged the population to make long hikes over rough and dangerous territory. It was common, despite the risk of running into an enemy patrol, for the people to trek five or six hours by the light of the full moon, all the way to the Lempa River to fish the familiar pools. When they had made it back, they made a celebration of feasting on tasty freshwater fish.

One day, Daisi, a very shy twelve-year-old health worker, brought me a plate of game hens, a special treat. As I was eating, she asked me if I liked them.

"Sure! They're delicious. Who caught them?"

"My brother. And how about the tortillas?"

"Really good," I lied. They were completely insipid.

"They're banana tortillas. We don't have any sorghum left."

"What do you mean? You're making tortillas from bananas?"

"Not the fruit, the tree trunk. Pretty awful, huh?"

As I finished what remained, I felt my heart aching with sadness and rage.

During a town meeting on one of my last days in El Jocotillo, Elizabeth's husband, the president of the PPL, asked me if I would give a little talk on health. What could I say? We all knew what was lacking most for better health care: our liberation. But in the meantime we had to try to solve some pressing problems: securing good drinking water, building latrines, improving our diet. The first two involved more than just a simple little speech. As for the third—what could I tell these hard-working people who clean and plant their corn fields with such determination, never knowing if they will be able to harvest the crop?

I decided to talk about the sources of vitamins and proteins available in the local game, like iguana or fish liver, as well as in wild fruits.

After I had talked a while, Chepe, a member of the local people's committee, asked me, "Lemons don't provide anything, do they?"

I was surprised; I hadn't realized people held lemons in such disdain. I explained what little I knew about the benefits of citrus fruits, fomenting a heated discussion between those who considered lemons too sour for the sick and for nursing mothers, and those who told of having drunk lemonade while nursing with no ill effects.

"That's what's so beautiful about this revolution," said Chepe, as he brought the meeting to a close. "We're always learning something new. I didn't know any of this stuff you've told us, Paco. Thanks."

Most of those present understood what I had said, but I still had to learn that a few discussions were not enough to change deeply-ingrained ideas and habits. Although it is true that the ability to internalize everything that is validated by experience is the bottom line for survival in the midst of armed aggression, nevertheless biases about health are so deeply rooted that it will be impossible to win the fight against them without a long-term educational process which will impel the people themselves to change.

Combat in the Intestinal Zone

"Good morning, sir," said Veronica, one of the new health workers. "What do you have for the flu?"

"I have some tetracycline. It's very good," I answered. "How much would you like?"

"I guess you know best. Give me two pesos' worth."

As part of a workshop in El Sicahuite, we were improvising a little theater piece to summarize the week's classes, on the use of antibiotics in bacterial and viral infections.

Eight of the nine health workers who had come into my "pharmacy" bought tetracycline for the flu. Some of them had hesitated, but I used strong arguments—"I know what I'm talking about because I learned this at school." To my disappointment, I had ended up convincing them.

This little socio-drama was a very useful exercise which allowed me to measure what had been assimilated and what needed to be reviewed. I decided to repeat the whole class, and we went over the dangers of antibiotic misuse once more.

Nonetheless, on returning to the tiny village a few weeks later, while conversing with Maclovia, the head health worker, I noticed a practically empty quart bottle of chloramphenicol. Maclovia looked away, embarrassed. She had been giving it to children with diarrhea.

"But why did you do that? We only use it in typhoid cases. It's really dangerous for kids. I'm sure you know that."

"I know, you're right. But the people are so insistent, and since we don't have any anti-diarrhetics, I figured this way, at least I would be killing off some germs."

Maclovia had been one of my best students. It was clear to

me that if I couldn't find a better way to spell out the effects and dangers of antibiotics, the people's habits of pill-popping, combined with social pressure, would always end up neutralizing the ideas I was trying to introduce.

Tetracycline had been so widely promoted that the people thought of it like aspirin, taken for headaches or an upset stomach; for the flu, people took it two or three times a day, depending on what they could afford. In their minds, the best drug was definitely tetracycline; ampicillin was no good, but penicillin would do in a pinch.

What could I do to counteract these bad habits? How could I make my explanations easier to understand so that they would sink in?

In the beginning, in order to simplify things, I had avoided talking about such essential matters as the importance of the intestinal flora and the damage done to it by antibiotics. I had only mentioned bacteria as causing infections. How could I illustrate the flora's biochemical role and the significance of its depletion when antibiotics are administered? I spent a long time going over different aspects of peasant life, searching for an appropriate image. Suddenly, it came to me. Since these peasants lived in the middle of a people's war, why not explain this business of the flora and the antibiotics in war terms, which were all too familiar to everyone?

So I got down to work. The "battle of the germs" eventually became an ideal method of communicating ideas essential to our work. But first terminology had to cease being an obstacle.

I translated anatomy into the rural vernacular, adapting the words the peasants used for the body parts of common farm animals: pigs, cows, and chickens. If I said the word "stomach," they took it to mean the whole abdomen, so we settled for "belly" and "gut" to differentiate between the stomach and the intestine. In a similar fashion, we adapted their vocabulary for other body parts and fluids: bile, throat, neck, and so on.

However, I had significantly less success in explaining the difference between one gut which was large and stationary and the other which was small and movable. Contrary to what was

in a hospital, civilians had no way of observing both
es during abdominal surgery.
   ne day in a workshop in Tequeque, we got a chance to clarify these language barriers and gain a better understanding of the "battle of the germs."

When the enemy started launching heavier and more frequent attacks on Chalatenango, the Subregional Council and the local popular committees (PPLs) decided to butcher one head of cattle in each municipality so the children could eat meat. The measure would also save the livestock from falling into enemy hands in case of a *guinda*.

At dawn, members of the health and education commissions began the slaughter. By the time I got there, they had already collected buckets of blood to use later in preparing blood-sausage. The atmosphere was festive.

"Before the war, when there was butchering to be done, I was the one they always called on," Henry, the local representative in charge of the operation, stated proudly. He was blind in one eye and was always seen wearing an old beat-up hat made from wicker. "I got my part of the beast, and in my house, we never had any lack of meat. But it's been more than two years since my last job."

Rubí, a health worker from a neighboring hamlet, was the first to arrive for the class I was improvising. She had a fifth grade education and was a quick learner. Politically she was very conscious, perhaps because one of her brothers was a member of the Vanguard Units and her sister was one of the best lay nurses we had in the hospital. Rubí would have been working at the hospital too, were it not for a hip deformity which caused her considerable difficulty in moving about. Personally I hoped that within another year, with a little more practical experience and maturity—she was only fifteen—she would be able to take over as the municipal health supervisor.

The PPL representatives were already skinning the animal when Beto, Toña and Rosa joined us. Toña and her nine-year-old son walked to class everyday from Patamera, where she was the village health worker. She was twenty-eight and lived with her parents, having split up with the boy's irresponsible father, despite people's comments and reproaches; I was particularly struck by this, since she was very shy and reserved. Her tenacity for learning made me especially fond of her. Like so many other peasants, she could write, that is to say, she could copy, but then she couldn't read her notes. When we jotted down the essential points covered in class, she made painstaking efforts to write it all down and in the afternoons, would review the material with Rubí's help. She confided to me that once the workshop was over, she was going to sign up for the adult literacy classes, and then she would be able to read for herself what she had copied down.

Toña was always the last to understand in class. When trying to answer my questions, her expression took on a strange mixture of concentration, willpower, and shyness. She was conscious of her deficiency but managed to laugh at herself and her frequent setbacks.

The rest of the class arrived after the animal was completely skinned. Fernando from Tequeque; Lito from San Antonio; Aminta and Beti from San Juan. At first we talked more about meat than anatomy, but when the abdomen was opened up, we got down to business.

I took hold of the small intestine and to everyone's amusement, demonstrated how it jiggled. Henry grabbed the end of the small intestine just below the belly and used a piece of corn husk to tie off the duodenum so nothing would spill out. He then pulled it out so we could see the shape and position of the large intestine. The health workers and the *compas* from the PPL crowded around, listening with interest as I lectured.

Fernando mentioned that they called the large intestine the "air gut."

"So what do you call the small one, then?"

"The water gut."

Henry seized the chance to illustrate the lesson Fernando was giving me.

"We'll cut it open to clean it, then you can see what we're talking about."

He grabbed the duodenum and cut off the corn-husk cord, letting some of the contents spill out.

...here, you see? This one's really watery. But here," he ...the large intestine, "there's just air in between the ...of... of..., well, of shit."

Everybody burst out laughing.

"In a pig, it's even easier to tell the difference between the two guts."

Henry's demonstration and plain talk illustrated perfectly what I had so laboriously been trying to explain in class.

Using this as the base, I then lectured on the function of the intestine, taking a piece of the organ to study its texture and observing how the contents became more and more solid as it approached the anus. It was easy now to see where the bile mixed with and colored the substances from the belly. With such a clear reference, everybody came to an easy understanding of the process of decomposition and assimilation of foodstuffs in the digestive tract.

In future classes, even when there was no animal to illustrate the material, my explanations greatly improved. Fernando and Henry's lesson, along with the new terms "air gut" and "water gut," made them more comprehensible.

The morning after that lesson, I got up earlier than usual to search for some visual aids to use in the next class. I found a broken roofing tile near the house where we held the classes and broke it into little pieces. I collected some pebbles, and picked a few chili peppers, half of them green and the other half already overripened and red.

When the *compas* saw the strange collection of objects on the table, Fernando was the first to ask the question on all their minds: "What is all this for?"

"No lecture today. We're going to stage a pretend battle in order to understand the effects of antibiotics better. Picture the center of the table as the inside of the intestine. The green chili peppers are the healthy bacteria, and the red ones represent bad germs that cause infection. The pieces of tile are parasites and the pebbles, viruses."

I told them to imagine that the intestine was a battle field in the controlled zones. The green chili peppers represent the *compas*. The red chili peppers would be the enemy invading with tanks—the parasitic tiles. The viruses, or pebbles in this case, were special armored cars, against which we had no weapons.

To illustrate a healthy intestine, all around the table we scattered green chili peppers, or good bacteria, the "*compas*" of the intestinal flora, with just a few tiles and red chilis as "infiltrators," which were kept under control by the strength of the flora.

"When there's an invasion—an infection, that is—the intestine fills up with red chilis, or bad bacteria. If we start to mortar-fire with tetracycline, what happens? Who dies?"

I tossed a tetracycline capsule on the table. The *compas* stared at me in awe.

Rosa spoke up. "The chili peppers. Both red and green."

"Right! Both are vulnerable to the shock wave and the shrapnel. What happens to the armored vehicles and the tanks?"

"Nothing." Fernando was catching on.

Next we took the case of an enemy harassment, a common incident. The battlefield displayed a few red chilis as the attacking force, in amongst the green.

"If we mortar again, what happens?"

"Both the red and the green will die again," said Lito.

"In equal numbers?"

" No. More green chili peppers . . . I mean, *compas*. There are more of them."

"What should we do, then?"

"Well, we should just let the ground troops handle it; maybe a well-placed grenade could do the job."

"Which antibiotic would we use as a grenade?"

Lito thought for a moment.

"Well, penicillin might do."

"And erythromycin, too," added Rubí.

We went on to stage a viral infection by invading the green chili peppers with pebbles. Rosa suggested that we fight back with penicillin grenades. What would happen? Who would die? Rosa had to think about it.

"Penicillin won't do any good there," said Fernando, adding jokingly, "The best thing we can do is go on a *guinda*."

"That's right! We have to preserve our forces. That's what we do on a *guinda*, isn't it? So now, in medical terms, how can we make a *guinda*?"

"Rest."

"Drink fruit juice."

"And what happens to the virus? It lays off, just like that?"

"Sure, exactly like the enemy! They can't take it for more than a week," exclaimed Toña.

We spent the whole morning like that, laughing, simulating different combat situations, doing "weapons" tests, and discussing their efficiency and viability in each case. From the moment in which health care took on such a familiar form, things had become unquestionably clearer.

"What happens if we fire a mortar or toss a grenade before the attack begins?"

"The enemy digs down in its trenches and casements just waiting for us. They're forewarned and they can hold out longer."

"And our attack? Can we win?"

"No, we're fucked."

"Exactly. If we use antibiotics for just any old thing, that's what happens. The enemy becomes more resistant."

Several months after the course had ended, I visited Toña in Patamera. She told me about a *compa* who often showed up to borrow the tooth-extracting equipment.

"And he always asks me for a few Bactrim or ampicillin, as well. One day I asked him why he needed them, and he told me it was to prevent an infection. Should he be doing that?"

"Some people do, although it isn't necessary if you do a clean job in the first place."

"That's what I told him. I said that it was a mistake because he'd just be killing off the '*compa*' bacteria, the good ones. He stared at me like I was crazy or something. Huh! He can laugh but I won't forget that lesson, ever."

Can't You See This Is an Operating Room?

Our column was exhausted after a hard, day-long march. Night was falling, but before we rested we still had one more damned peak to climb on a barely visible path that twisted its way through the six foot high grass. The only other vegetation in sight was a scattering of pine trees way up on the all too distant summit.

The enemy was invading the controlled zones, and we were marching with a detachment of the people's army to oppose the attack. It was my first experience of an enemy offensive. Up until then, all I knew were the impressive stories of past *guindas*, already legendary amongst us, named for the months in which they took place. May, October, and November were those in which the enemy siege had been broken, almost without using a single gun, each at very high cost. Dozens of civilians had been massacred in streams and riverbeds. Now fear and hunger filled the air. I think we were all tense. Would things go all right for us in this offensive or would it be another tragedy? One thing was sure. This was going to be a real test for our little Medical Surgical Unit (MSU).

It was pure luck that José, the party representative for the health sector, found me when he woke us up at 4 A.M. I had just come in the day before from a workshop I was giving to the local health workers in El Sicahuite.

"Wake up and get your pack ready. You're going on a mission."

"What? And the workshop? They're waiting for me," I protested. I hadn't yet gotten used to following orders without question, as military life demands.

"Forget the workshop. We've got an emergency on our hands. You're going with the MSU."

When I was ready, Jaime, the lay nurse in charge of the MSU, handed me a liter of IV fluid and a few surgical supplies to put in my backpack. Three other lay nurses, María, Arelí, and Clara, would be coming with us to round out our team; that's all there was to the MSU.

When José asked us if we had everything, neither Jaime nor I knew what to say. We'd never been on an MSU mission before.

Jaime showed me the list. It seemed really short on supplies, but José put an end to our complaints. "Now listen, that's the best we can do. Almost nothing's gotten through in the last few months."

I asked then which doctor was going with us. José looked at me straight in the eyes. "Don't worry about that. Jaime will take care of it," he said imperiously, in that typically mysterious tone military people use to talk about secrets, but which, for a novice like me, was merely annoying.

We set out and walked uphill for two hours before coming to a sudden halt. "Who are we waiting for?" I asked. Getting no response to my question, I began to understand that I had to control my curiosity. Pretty soon we saw some *compas*. One of them had marked European features—a tall, thin, aging man with sparse, fine, very white hair. It was soon apparent to me that this was Jordano, the doctor we were waiting for.

He gave us a perfunctory "hello" and began asking a litany of questions: Where would we be operating? When would the wounded arrive? Where was the fighting? What kind of supplies did we have? Did we have certain kinds of sutures, clamps, and emergency drugs? Jaime just calmly responded to all his questions: "No, no, we don't have any," or, "We don't know that." The old guy had been on the Front only ten days and was aghast at what he was finding. Nor could he have imagined that several hours of hard march were still awaiting him today. Shortly we were underway.

That evening, putting one foot in front of the other again and again, we finally reached the top of that damn hill, as the sky darkened prematurely and big black clouds announced rain.

A whole detachment and some of the Chiefs of Staff had preceded us, so dinner—cold beans and tortillas—was ready when we got there.

It started raining in sheets, a typical tropical downpour. Jaime, María, and I made a feeble attempt to shelter ourselves under our plastic ground cloth. We tried filling our canteens from the rivers of water that streamed down the folds in the plastic, but we were more successful at getting ourselves soaked than in collecting water.

Once the rain stopped, we tried to get some sleep, sharing one blanket between the three of us. For modesty's sake, María placed her pack between the two of us, leaving me almost completely exposed to the chilly mountain air. About an hour before dawn, weary of fighting such an invincible foe, I surrendered and got up. A thick-lipped, flat-nosed *compa* was standing guard on the summit, wrapped in one of those wonderful silk ponchos that Reagan sends us via the Salvadoran Army.

"Can't sleep, Paco?"

"It's too damn cold. I thought this was a tropical climate. Besides, I've never slept so completely at the mercy of the elements before."

"Oh, yeah. I didn't sleep a wink my first time either. But you get used to it. Before you know it you'll be sleeping on roots, rocks, any shitty old spot and you'll think it's goose down."

The man inspired me with confidence and seemed capable of great understanding. The night before I had watched as he mingled with the troops and the lay nurses, smiling as he peered through his thick glasses. Only when he told me his name was Arnoldo, did I realize that this humble man, taking his turn at guard duty, was a member of the Chiefs of Staff, in charge of health and logistics. He was my boss.

We stopped talking and turned to look towards the south, to the huge carpet of lights that was metropolitan San Salvador. It was eerie seeing the city so close. Each time that view sprawled out before us, we felt even more acutely the need to see the day when we would march into the Plaza Libertad.

From the east, little by little, the dawn's glow snuffed out the city lights. Yes, life might be hard, but it was also as splendid as the silhouette of the black mountains sketched on the crimson horizon. But the serenity was short-lived.

Within a few hours, our troops were already clashing with the enemy on top of a big mountain, known as La Montañona. We spent most of the day in the trenches, grateful that there were no wounded to treat. By the afternoon, the sounds of combat died down and our makeshift base camp under the pines was soon filled with enemy soldiers who had surrendered.

The prisoners were rapidly besieged by young guerrilla fighters, who traded their worn-out clothes for the captives' fancy jungle-print uniforms, compliments of the Pentagon. Groups of *compas* bargained with each of the twenty-five prisoners for their shirts, pants, or boots while, at the same time, they collected M-16 rifles, grenades, backpacks, canteens, M-79 grenade launchers, and other materiel.

I didn't doubt that the treatment we reserved for prisoners was humane and correct, but I was surprised by how relaxed the atmosphere was. The enemy soldiers didn't even have their hands tied, and a few greeted the *compas* familiarly, this being the second or third time they had surrendered.

"We couldn't surrender until the lieutenant got killed. He was a hard-liner and said that he would shoot anyone who gave up," one of the captured soldiers explained.

A little later, some *compas* brought in an eighteen year old with a slight injury, a clean bullet wound between the thumb and index finger of the right hand. Jordano treated it, giving the youth a few stitches.

"This is nothing to worry about," Jordano told him. "Ten days and you'll be good as new," he said, and with his index finger, squeezed the trigger of an imaginary gun.

The *compas* who had brought him in burst out laughing. "He's not a *compa*, man! He's a prisoner!"

The next day heavy fighting started at dawn. Hoping to strike our positions, planes dropped rockets and bombs all over the pine slopes. We realized that, contrary to the previous day, we would probably need someplace to operate and access to water. We were deciding what to do when the first casualty was brought in by members of his own squadron. A rocket had exploded right next to him, lodging a piece of shrapnel in his abdomen. The young man's name was Joaquín. He didn't look too bad off, since he was still able to talk, and didn't seem to be in great pain.

Jordano examined him closely: the fragment had entered his left side, under the ribs near the navel. María took his blood pressure, which was still relatively normal. Upon finishing the examination, however, Jordano looked concerned. He took Jaime and me aside to tell us that we had to operate as soon as possible. The shrapnel had penetrated Joaquín's abdomen and it was very likely that his spleen was ruptured. At that news, Jaime ran off to notify the command post of the situation.

"But how are you going to operate without a scrub nurse or anaesthetist? You don't even have any retractors."

"I know, it's rotten, but we've got to try. That's all we can do." We went about starting Joaquín on an IV.

Suddenly we heard the Chief of Operations yelling: "MSU! Withdraw from the area! That means *now!* " The enemy was closing in.

Things started moving really fast. We didn't have hammocks to carry the wounded or machetes to improvise splints for the fractured legs of two *compas* that had just come in. Who knows how we did it, but we soon found ourselves on the other side of the mountain, treating the victims of a real bitch of an air raid.

Among the seriously wounded was a *compa* with a lung full of blood, due to a chest injury. Jordano began searching for a thick tube to use for draining; a nasogastric tube seemed most appropriate for getting the air and blood out in order to restore negative pressure in the lung, thereby allowing it to reexpand and compress the bleeding vessel.

Jordano was pessimistic. This method could only work if we raised the patient some three feet off the ground, so that a recipient could collect the draining blood. It was a question of physics—without this difference in levels, the drainage wouldn't work. So I took a knife and started digging a hole where we could put a canteen, the only receptacle we had at hand. Nearby, part of the logistics team was watching us, as much aghast as distressed. One of them, whose city clothes implied that he had recently arrived on the Front, helped me start the boy on an IV.

We emptied the first canteen-full of blood. Jordano remained uneasy.

"That's an important vessel to be bleeding like that. In any other circumstances, I'd already be operating on him, but here it doesn't make any damn sense. The *compa* with the spleen injury is a priority. We can still help him."

Once more I emptied the canteen. And again and again. The strained faces of the logistics men looking on mirrored the tension of the situation. Although they had no real knowledge of medicine, they understood perfectly well what was happening. It wasn't the first time for them. When the *compa* died, they buried his body in a nearby trench which had been half washed out by the rains.

"Death made him look like such an old man, but, imagine, he was only seventeen," one of them whispered.

Finally we received permission to operate at a place a couple of hours walk away—all downhill. The *compas* from logistics carried the wounded along the steep, rocky, narrow path. Maneuvering downhill is the worst; all the weight falls on the front bearer, pushing him irremediably forward. The person at the rear feels like he is being dragged the whole way, adding to the danger of tripping or falling. The swaying of the hammock furthers the instability, increasing the risk of dropping the patient altogether.

But we soon reached a half-destroyed house, used by the detachment as a kitchen, and quickly converted it into a miniature campaign hospital. In one room, most of the roof was still intact, so that became the ward where we placed the wounded, directly on the earthen floor, reserving the two rope beds for the most serious cases. One of these beds was soon transformed into a makeshift operating table.

In order to take advantage of the daylight, we set up shop outside under a *guanacaste* tree. A twelve foot square perimeter around the operating table was declared the OR. We improvised a table for the surgical instruments with two boards and, on a nearby stone wall, laid out the other necessary materials.

Before we did anything else, we had to sterilize the instruments. We would need to put them in a closed tin container, and in turn, put that into a pot of boiling water. While some *compas* were off washing the instruments, I negotiated with the cooks for some space at their fires.

"You've got a lot of work, but I've got mine too," was the answer I got from Mayra, the head cook. "We have to get out some 400 tortillas for each meal. And when the *compas* from logistics come to pick them up, they damn well better be ready. The *compas* are out there fighting, you know."

We reached an agreement by taking some smoldering logs to start another fire.

"This is the first time I'm working the kitchen and the MSU at the same time," Mayra protested with a pleasant smile.

We divided up the work: Jaime would be the surgeon's assistant; María, the scrub nurse, with help from Arelí; Clara would look after the rest of the patients. I was petrified upon being assigned to anaesthesia, since the most I had ever done during an operation was to take vital signs.

"How much ketamine should I give him?" I asked Jordano.

"How the hell should I know? The anaesthetist always took care of that."

I recalled that the time when I had helped out, the anaesthetist administered the drug using a three cc syringe. But ketamine comes in three different concentrations.

"Well, what we've got here is the lowest concentration, so just give him three ccs and we'll see what happens," Jordano advised.

By then it was really late, almost 6 P.M. and Joaquín, the wounded *compa*, had been bleeding internally all day long. There was only about a half hour of daylight left, and all we could count on in the dark would be three flashlights with really low batteries. At the last minute, a *compa* produced a precious pair of brand new batteries. "Fucking A, man, terrific!"

Jordano was impatient. He started to put on his surgical gloves and asked María to watch closely because, on top of everything else, she had to learn to put her own on without contaminating them. The first time she tried, she inadvertently brushed her blouse, making the gloves unusable. We only had one pair left. Jordano explained the procedure to her again; following him step by step, this time she got it right.

María laid out the operating equipment on the "instrument table." The miserable collection included six hemostats, two anatomical clamps, two surgical clamps, a scalpel holder, and a suture holder. It was nowhere near enough for major surgery. There were no long hemostats, field clamps, retractors, intestinal clamps, or any of the other instruments normally required to do exploratory abdominal surgery. And as if things weren't bad enough, the scalpel didn't fit the only holder we had, so Jordano had to hold it with one of the hemostats.

"This is going to be a bloody mess," Jordano complained.

My anaesthetic supplies were equally paltry. Two or three bottles of ketamine, a couple of vials of atropine and diazepam; syringes and a blood pressure gauge, but no stethoscope; no corticosteroids or muscle relaxants; not even an ambu-bag or endotrachial tubes.

I administered the first dose of ketamine and we put Joaquín to sleep for the operation that had been so desperately delayed. Jordano spread sterile field sheets on the boy's naked abdomen. Since there weren't any clamps to hold them, he had to stitch them directly to the skin.

Joaquín practically leaped right off the table with the first stitch and almost tore off the field sheets. The others held him down, while I nervously administered a second and then finally a third dose.

Jordano explained his procedures to María so that she would learn the names of the different instruments and their function. When the incision had been made, Jaime used his gloved hands as retractors to hold the belly open.

The bed that we were using as the operating table was so

low that Jordano had to bend way over to see what he was doing. We didn't have surgical robes, so he worked bare chested. We all used red handkerchiefs over our mouths as surgical masks and didn't worry about head coverings.

"Who needs a surgical cap anyway," joked Jordano to everyone's amusement; he was practically bald.

A small crowd of spectators gathered around the "operating room," bewildered and slightly disconcerted by all our shouting and wild gestures. As the operation progressed, they slowly crept closer, crossing the imaginary boundary we had established.

Jordano reprimanded them. "Get out! Can't you see this is an operating room!?"

We all doubled over laughing, while the *compas* stared at us as if we were crazy. Understanding the absurdity of a situation can sometimes be so relative!

One of the onlookers was called over to hold a flashlight. He was obviously affected by what he saw. "Good God! It's just like butchering a pig!"

Jordano had been right about the spleen being ruptured and since this was the critical moment, he ordered everyone to pay close attention. "Don't move that light! Make sure the anaesthesia is deep enough! Have those instruments ready!" It was very tense work. Jordano, swearing like crazy, performed quickly and precisely. What a pro that guy was! Once the spleen had been removed, he looked up. "OK, if he's hung on this long, he'll make it now, in spite of the botched-up job we've had to do."

He cleaned out the cavity with previously boiled water and made sure there was no other damage. Joaquín's blood pressure improved rapidly. I felt a flood of relief.

Closing the incision was a long, difficult process since we didn't have any muscle relaxants. Joaquín was resisting, even in his anaesthetized sleep, and repeatedly burst the stitches.

There was some confusion when it came time to hand Jordano the sutures; the lay nurses got flustered by the unintelligible mixture of Dutch, French, and German on the envelopes and kept mixing them up. Jordano lost his patience and ended up pointing them out with his elbow, in order not to risk contaminating his surgical gloves: "Not that one—here, this one."

After six weary hours, we were done. It looked like Joaquín would pull through after all.

Our audience had already gone off to sleep. Even the lay nurses disappeared as soon as the operating room was more or less picked up. Jordano and Jaime checked up on our patient in "recovery," and then left to get some sleep, leaving me on call.

Having spent so much time with Joaquín, we had somewhat neglected the other patients. Between serious and light injuries, there were about twelve in all. I heard somebody groaning and went to see what was happening. The poor guy had a multiple fracture of his leg and worse, it was poorly immobilized. I felt horror and shame. How slow and inexpert we were!

The next day a number of members of the militia came to take the wounded to the hospital. Joaquín was apparently in stable condition, but Jordano was worried.

"That kid is pretty strong considering everything he's been through; but if he doesn't get a transfusion, he won't last the day. There's nothing but pure serum running in his veins."

Soon our attention was elsewhere. We went back into our operating room with another patient, Reyes. The little experience we had gained as a team helped us work much more effectively and efficiently this time.

But our joy was cut short when word reached us that Joaquín had died on arrival at the rear guard hospital. Somebody cried out, "Fuck this shit!," while the rest of us fell into that sparse silence with which news like that is always received.

A few days later we abandoned that site, evading a heavy enemy attack. This time we walked for thirty-six hours behind enemy lines and managed to outwit them, suffering only one minor casualty—a bullet in the fleshy part of a *compa's* butt.

After the retreat was over, we insisted on a meeting with the party representative, José, to evaluate the experience. We were adamant about several points: do whatever was necessary to get the materials needed to make fresh blood transfusions;

have the equipment and supplies on hand at all times for a MSU to face any emergency. But most of all we criticized him for sending six greenhorns, none of whom had previous MSU experience. We knew only too well that Joaquín and the youth with the chest injury had paid a terrible price for all these shortcomings.

José defended his decision, arguing that there had been no other health personnel available during the emergency. It was the cruel reality, part of the unequal conditions in which this war is waged.

But José, sensing our sadness, added, "Well, you've had your trial by fire. It's a bitch, but that's how you learn here, even if pain and death unfortunately have to be all too much part of it." Then he looked right at me, and said, "Just wait. You'll be one of the best damn anaesthetists the people's war has seen."

We Went Up into the Hills Thinking We'd Be Back Home in a Couple of Weeks

Bernardo, as a surgeon, when and where did you join the guerrillas?

Right at the end of 1980, when we were getting ready for the January 10, 1981, offensive. I was assigned to the Felipe Peña Front, which is part of the Modesto Ramírez Central Front.

Which subregion were you in?

It was called "Naranja," near Tenancingo. In those days, that front was very different from now. Each subregion was nothing more than a tiny area completely surrounded by enemy outposts. This one, even at its widest part, took only three hours to cross on foot. It was pretty flat, with just a couple of big hills.

What was the health picture there?

Extremely precarious. Theoretically, we were supposed to have a central hospital and several campaign medical stations, but there was nothing like that. We had to start from scratch, organizing and training people. That's what I did from the moment I arrived. We had our first experience with combat wounded on New Year's Day, even before the start of the offensive.

Were you the only doctor in the subregion?

Yes. I relied heavily on the peasants. We gave twenty-one people a crash course in basic field medicine; it lasted a total of three weeks, not counting time out for combat and *guindas*.

None of them had ever participated in any kind of surgery. I was sure there were going to be lots of problems. This was indeed confirmed that New Year's night; problems with the anaesthetist, the scrub nurse, the surgeon's assistant, problems all over the place.

There were no other medical professionals—just you?

During the first couple of months of 1981 there were a number of other doctors and paramedics working in different subregions, but they didn't last long. The doctors who joined up at that time believed the war wouldn't last more than two months or so. Most of us got involved thinking we'd be back home and at work in a couple of weeks. The majority left in a few months. The Felipe Peña Front takes in three zones: the area around Cinquera, the Guazapa volcano and its surroundings, and a small region on the the other side of the Troncal del Norte Highway. By mid-1981, this whole front was left practically without medical professionals, just one sixth year medical student and one doctor.

You, right?

Yes. We had to work hard training people in a lot of different areas, including nursing. We managed to train some very competent lay nurses, who later became OR scrub nurses. We also worked on making bandaging materials, rounding up whatever old clothes or rags we could find in deserted villages and turning them into dressings, swabs, and compresses.

We spent a lot of time that first year teaching people how to handle anaesthesia. We finally got to the point where the patients were effectively anaesthetized, working with drugs that they still don't use even in Chalatenango.

How did you manage that?

We intubated the patients and maintained them with a drop system, connected behind the ambu-bag with a device we designed right there on the front. That allowed us to use different kinds of drugs, like muscle relaxants: tubocurarine, succinylcholine, Pavulon, and so on. Plus, we administered inhalant anaesthesia like halothane, penthane, or fluothane, combined with ketamine, all widely used in modern medicine. All of this made operating easier. Some of these people we trained eventually got to be pretty good, given the circumstances, and formed the base of technicians for the hospitals and MSUs.

We were particularly interested in training peasants as surgeon's assistants; as part of the course, we would operate on dogs, pointing out muscular tissues, organs, and blood vessels. Before long, these trainees were able to anticipate certain needs and had a working knowledge of the operational sequence.

In the process, we were able to get rid of the notion that the least adequate persons should be assigned to health. We fought hard to get the best, most willing *compas* for our work, those who were really eager to learn.

Under what conditions did you operate?

You might call it "surgery in motion." It was actually kind of funny. The enemy would show up daily at about 9 A.M. Normally the alarm sounded and we had ten minutes to get out of camp. But when we had to operate, we would wait until 10 A.M. to see if there was really going to be an attack or not. If there was no action by then, we would go ahead with our plans. Sometimes the enemy wouldn't come until later, which meant we had to run off into the hills with the patient heavily anaesthetized.

I remember one time we were closing a urinary fistula—the urethra had been ruptured near the testicles by a bullet. It was a very delicate operation with little chance of success. We had barely closed the fistula when we had to flee, with the urinary catheter just hanging there, open-ended. Miraculously, the *compa's* urethra healed within six weeks.

For days and weeks on end, we had recuperating patients hidden in isolated caves and gullies. It was a horrible situation. That's what happened to those who were wounded in Cinquera. As you know, we were hit harder there than usual. In fact, I never saw more wounded than in that engagement; not even in other major attacks, like the one on Cerrón Grande, did we have half as many. There were some sixty-odd injured *compas* in all, of which twenty or twenty-five were more or less serious cases.

Imagine taking care of a patient like Isaias in those

conditions.* A bullet hit him in the fifth left intercostal space and then went downward, damaging his lung, diaphragm, and intestine. There was a serious problem of sepsis and he went into shock. Once operated on, he came through with no major problems. But a fragment had damaged a nerve in the lower lumbar region, which still gives him trouble today. Nevertheless, we were able to repair the abdominal damage and control the sepsis, which otherwise would have killed him.

There were times when I had to do as many as five cases of abdominal surgery in twenty-four to thirty-six hours.

What did you think about having so much responsibility?

It's very complicated and rather difficult to explain. In people's eyes, you become bigger than life. You're no longer just anybody. You lose the right to be afraid, or at least, to show your fear in front of others. You bear the responsibility for the medical care of the entire population, as well as the burden of your own mental health. There's no shoulder around to cry on; you personally feel like you're getting smaller and smaller, as if you're carrying a great weight on your shoulders.

Did the reality which the doctors confronted greatly surpass their technical capacities and professional training?

Traumatic wounds in war are very different from those in civilian life. They're much more gory, more extreme, and, as a doctor, they traumatize you, too. There are moments when you feel completely inept: the lack of trained personnel and supplies and the uncertainty weigh heavily on you. When yet another life had slipped out of his hands, I recall seeing another of our doctors, Noé, break down, crying as a man and as a doctor. I knew exactly how he felt. That's what happens to you. Nevertheless, you're the last resource and you've got to live up to the situation. Your only hope is to try to do the very best you can.

There are some lives you just can't save without modern technology. Given the serious nature of some wounds, like a severed major artery, say, all you can do is watch death slowly take over. Uncertainty plays a big role. Maybe you're in combat, where there's not really much you can do. Other times,

---

*An interview with Isaias appears on pages 155–158.

the wounded don't get to you until it's already too late. Their limbs are destroyed, and they've practically lost all their blood, and in the end, they just glide into something like a tunnel. That is how I describe death. When someone starts dying, he starts gliding . . . gliding . . . dead.

Cranial wounds are another dilemma. Conditions for dealing surgically with them just don't exist on the war fronts. Sometimes they pull through, but then they usually are left with serious functional disabilities.

Did you ever think about what would happen if you were seriously injured?

Well, there was the time they started bombing us with 120mm mortars, just when we had almost finished evacuating the hospital for other reasons. One of the grenades fell right smack in the operating room. There was smoke and dust everywhere. I had been out in the patio and could hear someone crying inside. I ran in, found a *compa* who had been lightly wounded by the impact, threw him over my shoulder, jumped on a horse, and got the hell out of there. My shirt got covered in blood, so when I caught up with the others, they thought I had been wounded; before long, everyone was talking anxiously about what a disaster it would be if I were to get hurt. I always figured, well sure, my getting wounded would be a problem, not so much for me, but because where would they ever find another doctor to replace me?

Doctors Double as Architects

As we walked up and down, crossing rivers and climbing hills in that area known as the controlled zones of Chalatenango, the *compas* had a habit of pointing out important landmarks.

"That's where they massacred thirty-two civilians from my village."

"Here's where Laura fell in combat."

Former sites of hospitals were always mentioned.

"This is where it was in 1982 after the November *guinda*."

"It was here when we amputated Martín's leg."

How many hospitals have been set up only to be later packed up and relocated! The very nature of this war makes hospitals a prime enemy target, forcing us to move them constantly.

Paralleling the development of the people's army, medical care has evolved from the most elementary state to a greater level of sophistication. The army began with isolated groups of poorly-armed *compas*, but little by little, these grew until they formed the Vanguard Units, and later, brigades.

At first, the hospitals were located in isolated adobe huts; in time, we took over bigger dwellings and then whole groups of houses, creating "Guerrilla Hospital Complexes" where each area—logistics, the pharmacy, the sterilization unit, patients' and personnel quarters—had its own separate location. The best spot was always reserved for the operating room.

During the time I spent in the war, we began building hospitals hidden up in the hills, which meant that doctors were also called upon to become guerrilla architects. The progressive transformation of our operating rooms provides a good gauge of the development of our hospital facilities.

The first war zone OR I worked in was located in an earthen-floor adobe house. It had a large operating table and a smaller surface for the scrub nurse's use. Surgical supplies were kept on shelves mounted on the walls. Although this installation had been designed by a professional OR nurse, it was not without its problems: the table was too wide, making it difficult for the surgeon to get close to the patient, there was not enough access to daylight, and finally, no one respected the operating room as a restricted area.

The OR nurse tried to lay down the law by insisting that, other than for surgery, the area was off-limits. But in practice, she never succeeded. Because the OR was the only place in the whole hospital that was quiet and guaranteed a semblance of privacy, it was our favorite refuge. When she was transferred, with her went any regard for the orthodox definition of an operating room.

In that hospital and in others, the OR became alternately conference room, cafeteria, pantry, office, and dormitory. That it was only a restricted area during an actual operation didn't surprise anyone. Sometimes there wasn't even a door separating it from the ward.

The doctors in the hospital during this period didn't have much experience. A lot of them were fifth or sixth year medical students who had fled the repression. They had finished their studies in the mountains, where the practice they got facing new and difficult situations completed their training.

They didn't adhere to traditional concepts of surgical discipline. They just did everything they could to save a patient's life, almost without understanding how they succeeded. Indeed, style was the least important element: incisions were stitched together with little regard for aesthetics, leaving scars that were far too big; but these doctors believed in their lucky star and in the resilience of their patients, who for the most part were strong young men and women. When they found themselves faced with a damaged intestine, they concentrated on implementing the theory of resection, not worrying about the bits of grass or leaves that the mountain winds blew into the open abdomen; they simply reached in with their "sterile" gloves and picked the debris out. They certainly weren't going to be bothered by not having proper surgical robes and caps. Nor did they get upset when a peasant holding the flashlight spat on the floor. Despite all this, post-operative infections were quite infrequent, something that often puzzled many of us.

In fact, we only began to respect proper operating room discipline when some medical specialists started to enter the Front. At first, their requirements seemed exaggerated, especially Diana's.

Once while setting up a hospital in a house that was in good condition, we heard noise up on the kitchen roof. Soon, we saw pieces of adobe flying and could make out the sound of a machete, chopping at the bamboo poles supporting the roofing tiles.

Having just arrived on the Front, Diana, an orthopedic specialist, was set on having a perfect operating room, totally aseptic and properly illuminated. To insure this, she and Cirilo, the anaesthetist, had climbed up on the roof to open a skylight over the kitchen, which she had selected as the site best suited for her purposes. It made me furious to see those two tearing apart a house in such good shape; places like that were really hard to come by in the controlled zones. Not only that, but even with a skylight, the kitchen was so closed in that I was sure the heat would be unbearable inside. Before we could find out who was right, Diana, who had been nicknamed "Attila," thanks to this incident got transferred to another hospital, and we set up the operating room on the porch which met the necessary light and sanitary conditions for the surgery that we would be performing.

Nonetheless, Diana's reputation for being adamant about creating a well-enclosed OR for orthopedic surgery continued. Her new assignment was in a hospital codenamed "H-60," which everybody called "Hole 60" because of its location in a gully. An old rectangular water tank in the mouth of the ravine was used as the back wall of the new operating room; its other three sides were built from scrap materials found in Las Flores. Diana whitewashed and disinfected that room with lime and improved the lighting by installing windows taken from some of the best houses in the abandoned town.

This first of Diana's "ideal operating rooms" was abandoned just a few days after it was finished: the whole hospital had to be moved on account of an enemy incursion.

Diana resumed her project at the next location in the village of San Juan. This time, to guarantee asepsis, she decided to build on a spot beyond the other huts, under an avocado tree which provided shade and good protective cover from aerial detection.

The new OR was assembled from bamboo poles split down the middle. The ribbed walls helped to keep the sun out and, to some degree, to control the circulation of air, dust, and germs. Unfortunately, the rather appealing oriental atmosphere created by the bamboo construction had its drawbacks, for the walls were soon infested with bugs that chewed them away, leaving sawdust everywhere.

Yet that wasn't the only problem. The skylight, which in our circumstances was nothing more than an opening in the roof, provided good daylight, but also let in unfiltered air and dust. The only solution was to install a window; but where would we find one in such a poor part of the zone? Nothing was impossible for Diana. Accompanied by a few lay nurses, she explored the area until eventually they found a window big enough to do the job. The hitch was that they had to bring the new-found window all the way back from Las Flores, four hours' walk away.

The window was so heavy that the *compas* had to take turns carrying it on their backs along the overgrown, dusty, rock-strewn road. When they reached the Sumpul River they had to cross a bridge that the guerrillas had improvised after blowing up the first one in 1979. Treading its narrow length was not the only difficult obstacle to overcome. At the far side of the crossing, they had to scale a retaining wall as well.

But finally they did get there, exhausted. Happy and

relieved to unburden themselves of their cargo, they started to lean the window against one of the walls of the operating room.

Diana ran in with instructions. "Here: Lean it up against this pole. That's it—easy now."

As luck would have it, the *compa* who was helping to lower the damn thing, maybe on account of sweaty hands—or who knows why—lost his grip and we all watched helplessly as the precious load crashed to the ground. There was nothing else to do but laugh at first and finally gather up the larger pieces of glass and figure out how to salvage the project. We ended up with a significantly smaller skylight, yet that operating room was one of the best we ever built.

During this same period, we built a general hospital on the other side of the controlled zones in the village of El Tamarindo. The "El Tamarindo Hospital Complex" and the orthopedic hospital were our most ambitious achievements, architecturally and functionally speaking.

As mentioned before, the civilian population was usually very supportive of the task of constructing a new hospital. They also helped with digging trenches, carrying the wounded, and planting crops for provisions. But given the scale of this project, it was not realistic to rely solely on them, especially since it was now the planting season.

Jordano and I were in charge of organizing and supervising the construction. We suggested that some *compas* be reassigned from military duty to work on the site, but all we got was one person, Rigoberto, who then acted as the foreman overseeing the teams of civilians that came to pitch in during their free time.

Jordano drafted the plans. The operating room was the most strategic and urgent element, since once it was built, the hospital could open for business. It was still the dry season, so patients and staff would be able to sleep outside. The kitchen would be the second priority. It would be built Vietnamese style, using a long underground tunnel to create a draft and disperse the smoke that might otherwise betray our position to air reconnaissance.

Rigoberto was very proud of himself the day that the

operating room was finished. He pointed out how he had used very durable wood to construct the walls and had made them even higher than we had asked for.

When it came to the roof, we discovered less agreeable changes. We had wanted a three foot eave all around to keep the rain out, but what Rigoberto had produced was a roof that barely reached the outer wall.

"This isn't Paris or Amsterdam, you know," Rigoberto replied. "We don't make roofs like that here."

We explained that we had indeed seen this kind of overhanging eave here, and not in Europe, where there are no heavy tropical rains; but Rigoberto had already decided to make this a cultural conflict and he wasn't going to change his mind. When the rains came, we ended up having to close off the upper part of the OR, which we had initially left open for light and ventilation. This change considerably reduced the amount of available daylight.

Alfredo, the supply master and Felipe, an ex-prisoner who had been freed during the last attack by the *compas* on the town of Chalatenango, finished off the insides. They were both very resourceful.

We showed them a drawing of the ideal operating table, which easily converted itself into a stretcher to take the patient to the intensive care unit or back to the ward. We wanted the table top to be adjustable so we could either put the patient in a completely horizontal position for administering different kinds of anaesthesia—using the bubble in a vial of injectable medicine as a level—or, in the case of shock, change the angle so that the patient's feet would be higher than the head. Alfredo and Felipe caught on right away and went off to Las Flores to rummage through the materials there. We had no doubts that they would come through with something good, and they did.

Alfredo used his Chalatenango peasant's tradition to perfect the Vietnamese-style kitchen. He designed a very small opening for the hearth, building it out of earthen clay and organic matter, the mixture used to make bread-baking ovens, which retains heat while saving on firewood. He also found a large steel plate to use as a *comal*, the grill used for cooking tortillas. The cooks were delighted with its size because it allowed them to make lots of tortillas at once.

As soon as the operating room and the kitchen were ready, the hospital began to take patients. Everyone collaborated to finish the rest of the facilities. The lay nurses carried roofing tiles on their heads, and we all dug trenches for the defense system, a couple of feet more every day. We had to have everything ready before the pending attack on Cerrón Grande.

Although important planned attacks were usually well-guarded secrets, this one we all knew about. Only the enemy was caught by surprise, despite all its fancy intelligence equipment. The closer we got to the date, the harder we worked at preparations. We completed the hut which would be the ward for the more serious cases. We prepared bandages and compresses, sterilized equipment, checked the reserve supplies of medicines and serum, and finished making more bamboo cots for the patients.

The day before the attack, a group of civilians brought enough bamboo, vines, and sticks to make twenty-five new *tapexcos,* so that the ward would be ready to function. We were lucky, as it turned out, and didn't need them all. Just the same, we were happy and pleased at having been so well-prepared to meet any emergency. Now we could count on a first-class "Guerrilla Hospital Complex."

Learning All We Can

Mornings at our hospitals were devoted to activities common to any medical facility: workers preparing shots and medications or bringing patients breakfast plates of beans and tortillas, lay nurses combing patients' hair after bathing them.

But the afternoons were a very different story. Some of the lay nurses sat in circles with patients to study history, while over in another corner, others learned to read and write using a piece of an old broken blackboard, salvaged from a schoolhouse destroyed in an air raid. Still another group might be attending a workshop given by the doctors on nursing techniques or anaesthesia.

Literacy training was the most important of all. A lot of the lay nurses were illiterate; a number of them didn't even know how to tell time, which was especially awkward when it was their turn to be on night call, since they kept waking you up to see if their shift was over.

The reading classes were really appreciated, but for some reason, history and political education didn't provoke similar enthusiasm. We tried different ways of making them more interesting: we scheduled them for the morning when the mind is clearer, and we introduced new materials.

At one point, since there were only three of us who could give these lectures, we divided the hospital team into three groups. I was assigned to the supply and kitchen staff. We used a calabash, a big round squash, as a makeshift globe, and a flashlight for the sun; I explained what makes night and day, how volcanoes are formed, and how the earth is constantly changing. We drew a crude world map, marking the capitalist countries, the socialist states, and those nations struggling for their liberation. Many countries which the *compas* knew only from newscasts were located on our map, and we talked about their history.

Our group included some very different individuals. Alfredo and Felipe, the supply masters, were both middle-aged; Miriam, the cook, was young and vibrant; Rigo, the messenger-boy, was only fourteen. He enjoyed reading so much we dubbed him "Professor." However, most of the young girls in my group, and in the other two as well, yawned openly, doing nothing to hide their boredom. Was this due to the oppressive weight of a cultural inheritance that imposes political ignorance on women? Or was it just too hard to understand us and penetrate our abstract thinking? One thing was sure; whenever any of the wounded took part in the discussion, things became much more dynamic. They wanted to know about everything. Was this because they were men? Or was it because, as combatants, they felt directly affected by world politics?

In any case, the best talks were given by special guests, like Rutilio Sánchez, one of the most popular and best-loved persons on the Front.

The fact that Tilo was a priest figured greatly in the impact of this man, converting him into a kind of witch doctor, psychologist, poet, and activist all rolled into one. More than anything else, he knew how to inspire confidence in his people. They would never forget how, during the terrible *guinda* of November 1982, he had celebrated the Word, sharing fear and defying danger.

So when the staff and patients learned that this special priest would be speaking, everybody got excited. Mario, the doctor in charge, began somewhat pompously introducing him, but then Father Tilo broke in. "I'm not going to bore you with stuff you already know," he said. "Surely you've all been thinking a lot about this war, and you probably have some questions, too. Maybe I can try to answer a few of them."

One by one, the *compas* got up the courage to ask him about the state of the dialogue with the government, or about international support for our struggle. They also wanted to know about the importance of the Contadora process. Jaime asked if, after we had won the war, we would have to pay the debt that Duarte was accumulating in buying bullets and bombs to use against us. Tilo spoke about everything—or almost everything, since that time no one brought up religion.

Staff turnover was so frequent that the medical training courses became a never-ending process. In five or six months, a young woman could learn basic medical skills and then be assigned to work in a mobile unit. Somebody else would always show up to take her place.

One day Federico, an acupuncturist from the Felipe Peña Front, paid us a visit. He was going to acquaint us with this medical approach, which was new for most of us. The skeptics among us were quickly converted when he rapidly relieved the pain of a *compa* whose arm had been amputated. The peasants were receptive to the concepts behind this kind of medicine, but unfortunately, our course was interrupted by a *guinda* and never continued.

Jordano, who was in charge of professional development, aimed at meeting the doctors' need to increase their competence. Faced with such a demanding reality, we were all too aware of our obligation to constantly improve our technical level. As the most experienced surgeon on the Front, he gave an intensive course in surgery.

One of the most unusual educational activities was a symposium of doctors in the people's war, convened on the Felipe Peña Front. Nearly all the physicians from both fronts, along with the battalion health chiefs and a few lay nurses with broad experience, participated in the event, which was organized to synthesize the medical experiences of the previous five years. The meeting only lasted twenty days due to a *guinda* and the subsequent attack on Cerrón Grande, but both occasions provided an opportunity to put some of the conclusions already reached in the symposium into practice.

We devoted long discussions to the problem of transporting wounded from one front to another, and as a result decided to adopt several new measures. We realized we had to initiate self-help and mutual-help training among the troops, because our access to transport was severely limited. It was essential that the *compas* themselves learn to apply first aid, most of all to control hemorrhaging. So classes were started.

After the Cerrón Grande attack, during the transfer of patients to Chalatenango, we experimented for the first time with a halfway station, to deal with the seriously wounded who suffered most from the upheaval of being moved. It proved to be a clear success.

Another important discussion in the symposium centered on the location of the MSU and the different combat medical stations. We worked according to two criteria: the time needed to tend to serious wounds and the military measures necessary to allow us to do our job safely.

In order to do a proper evaluation, as well as to better define the tasks of medical and paramedical personnel, we realized we needed statistical data to determine which conditions increased our casualties and which raised the chances of a wounded *compa's* survival. The figures we gathered revealed an interesting fact. A relatively high number of squadron, platoon, and even detachment officers had been wounded in combat, a demonstration of the difference between a bourgeois army and a popular one, in which officers run the same risks as the rank and file soldiers.

All in all, we set up norms for internal medicine and for surgery, based on the practices which had proved to be effective and adequate in this people's war, leaving behind the theories of different schools of medical thought.

One educational initiative which proved to be particularly successful occurred in the hospital we built in El Tamarindo. Jordano proposed to train a lay nurse for intensive care handling for the first time.

We met with the head of the hospital to choose the candidate. We already had someone in mind: Rosario, a lay nurse who displayed a great eagerness to learn, despite having minimal experience. Jordano gave her private instruction, and we all admired how quickly she assimilated so much theory from him. Her practical experience eventually turned her into one of the best lay nurses on the Front.

Rosario was just beginning her career as an intensive care nurse when two *compas* with particularly ugly wounds were brought in. They had been injured by rockets from an Israeli-made 0-2 spotter plane. One of the victims, Garri, was wounded by a fragment that went through his thigh and came out between his legs, destroying his scrotum, but miraculously not damaging his testicles. Eusebio, the other *compa*, got hit in the face by a piece of shrapnel, which had completely destroyed his lips and left cheek and caused extensive nerve damage. Of the two of them, Eusebio's wounds gave Rosario the most challenging task.

A few months earlier we had to care for another *compa* who had suffered a similar injury, where facial wounds and damage to his palate had left him unable to ingest food. At that point, Jordano didn't know what the normal war surgery procedure in such cases was, but he opted for introducing a catheter into the stomach directly through the abdominal wall. By feeding the patient through the catheter, we bypassed his wounded mouth and thereby reduced salivation, which helped the healing process. The operation was such a complete success that we began to use it for all severe maxillo-facial wounds. We followed this procedure for Eusebio now.

Taking care of Eusebio meant a lot of work for Rosario. She had to use her knowledge of nutrition to prepare food for him, and then feed it to him through the catheter. His wounds required strict attention, his mouth had to be aspirated, and for the first few days it was also her job to keep a careful eye on the *compa's* endotrachial tube.

Another one of Rosario's patients was Carlos, a member of the Special Forces who, on the Felipe Peña Front, had more than seventeen feet of his small intestine removed; that is to say, nearly all of it. We knew he was a high risk patient when he arrived, but his stay in the hospital turned out to be much sadder and more difficult than anyone had ever imagined it could be.

Carlos was put on a special diet which, whenever possible, included milk and fish from Los Amates, three hours away. Cheese and eggs were sold in some villages bordering on the controlled zones, but travel to them depended on the military situation. More than once, the new patient had to settle for beans and tortillas, which helped neither his recovery nor his ability to resist infection. We were afraid that a *guinda* would kill Carlos.

We wanted to get him out of the Front, but to do so was always a critical operation, contingent on underground contacts which, along with prisoner exchanges, were infrequent and unpredictable. We knew the Red Cross wouldn't take on such a case, since they see their duty as taking care of the civilian population. In any case, they hadn't been entering the controlled zones. Government army actions had blocked them from providing any real services to civilians there.

The situation was desperate. Carlos was doomed to starve to death in the intensive care unit. I was no longer working at the hospital, but each time I came to visit, I found him weaker and thinner, and I felt a pang of guilt just for eating my ration of beans and tortillas. In spite of everything, his face reflected a calm, patient, tenacious fight against death. I don't know how he managed to resist. At times, his expression could be sad, afraid, or terribly lonely, but it was never desperate. It reminded me of what another patient, who had been on the verge of bleeding to death, had once told me, "I didn't waste my time with fear then. I just kept one thing in mind: that I was part of the struggle and, for the moment, the struggle was staying alive."

Finally, Carlos died. Life is never the same for someone who has watched a brother die like that. El Salvador is full of men and women like him. I don't know how Rosario experienced his agony; she isn't going to write a book. But I saw her covering him with the blanket she herself had washed and, when his strength had given out, I watched her talk him into eating, which was especially important since the only IV to be had was saline solution. I admired her as she bathed his naked, gray body, without forgetting his penis, never repelled by the smell of putrification which announced approaching death.

I have seen dedicated professional nurses in gloomy, modern hospitals working with terminal patients. But watching as Rosario, a fifteen-year-old peasant girl, nursed Carlos, I knew that these people were winning their struggle.

Not even at the Bethesda Medical Center, where they operated on Reagan, could anyone have provided him with equally humble, loving care.

A Letter from Carolina

The Felipe Peña Front, east of Chalatenango, has been characterized by constant government army incursions, but the regime's troops were never able to dislodge our forces nor impede our permanent presence in the area. What follows is abstracted from a letter I received from another doctor, Carolina, telling me about the joys and struggles of life as a battalion doctor there in late 1983.

As I crossed the Cerrón Grande reservoir, on my way from Chalate to Felipe Peña, I discovered that the biggest problem wasn't the enemy or the lousy boats that kept filling up with water, but rather the clouds of mosquitoes, so dense that they even blocked out the moonlight. I made it to the MSU an hour after reaching shore. There were two Medical Surgical Units then, one for each battalion. I was introduced to the people I would be working with for the next few months: the supply masters, the cook, the surgeon, the lay nurses, and the scrub nurse, Esmeralda, whom I liked right away.

We talked a lot together, Esmeralda and I. She confided to me that she was tired of being toothless, and she would love to be able to chew properly. She wasn't even twenty yet. She was on the verge of writing to her boyfriend Arturo in Chalate to tell him that this would be her last letter, because it was just too difficult to maintain a long-distance relationship in this war. She also told me how sick she was of working.

"Well now, Esmeralda," I told her, "there are times when we all feel bored, and times when. . . ."

"No, I really am bored," she insisted.

"Don't worry. Pretty soon we'll be going on a mission and that will change."

"Yeah, sure," she responded without conviction. "Hey, hold out your hand—here's a little flour with sugar."

"You always have some saved up?"

"No, not at all. Just the strategic reserve they gave us last week, that's all."

We kept on talking, our tongues partially paralyzed by the dry mixture, unconcerned about the day when this ration might really be needed.

When night fell there, instead of lighting fires, we always put them out. There was an enemy position on the hill in front of us. They could see us, and we could see them. Sometimes they would fire off a volley just for the hell of it. Other times they shouted at us with megaphones: "Hey kid, go back home. Your mother's waiting for you." "Turn yourself in . . . report to the base with your weapons." Now and then, helicopters dropped leaflets giving the prices they would pay for weapons brought in by those who surrendered. Or other times we could hear "Guerrillas . . . Faggots! Cocksuckers!"

Two weeks after that reservoir crossing I got malaria—tremors, chills, fever. After you've had it a few times, it's really nothing more than a bad flu. Esmeralda took care of me in my hammock. Before long we got word that in two days we were to leave on a mission. That was just barely time enough for me to get back on my feet.

On the designated day, in the middle of a large natural clearing under the setting sun, our battalions were joined by those of the FAL (one of the five parties composing the FMLN). There were so many familiar faces! We all started greeting one another, laughing. Soon I began to feel a nervous knot in my stomach but the detachment chiefs called roll, and before I knew it, those of us from the MSU fell in with the service unit. Most of the women in the outfit wore outrageously colored skirts, red, pink, purple—and only a few made the "mistake" of wearing olive green. They carried gourds strapped to their backpacks and M-16's slung over their shoulders. Everyone complained about how heavy the packs were.

"Attention!"

We lined up without a word, counting off: "One! Two!

Three! . . . Eight and last! Column closed!" Whenever somebody goofed, we would make a scene laughing.

We all quieted down when Commander Ramón, the chief of the brigade, briefly explained the military and political importance of the mission. We sang the FPL hymn and then, together with the *compas* from the FAL, the "International."

When we got going, I could barely manage with all the weight. My chest hurt and I felt like I wouldn't be able to continue. Was it psychological or due to the malaria? I felt as if my lungs would explode. I turned red, then yellow, but I didn't stop. Some *compas* took my pack, telling me not to worry about it; and though I consider myself a proud and strong-willed woman, who could never let a man carry anything for me, I said, "Thanks, *compa*. I just can't do it."

The service platoon included logistics and kitchen crews, which meant that as we advanced, the huge iron pot used to cook the corn for tortillas banged against the rocks, broadcasting our passing. It was a moonless night. Since I had trouble following Esmeralda in the column, I picked up a glowworm and hung it on her pack, which helped guide me as she advanced in front of me.

"Don't anybody get lost!" came the order from the head of the column, relaying its way along the human chain.

"A hole on the right . . . on the right, a . . . Ah!"

"Keep quiet and get down . . . quiet and. . . ."

"Keeping moving . . . Keep moving. . . ."

After marching for several hours, the service unit separated from the combatants and we continued on our own. Soon we got lost in some godforsaken place. Full of stones and thorny, scratchy branches, it was even darker than where we had been walking before. Our confusion caused a tremendous uproar. The iron pot clanged like a church bell against almost every rock. At first, the *compas* whispered, but gradually their voices grew louder and, before long, it was pure bedlam.

"Turn back!" the order finally came, to our great relief.

Each of us got out as best we could. I only managed thanks to the glowworm. It was so dark at times, I didn't know if my eyes were open or not. Finally, crawling on all fours, scraped and bruised, we made it back to the road.

We reached a house, where we received permission to rest. I lay down next to Esmeralda, who had already spread out her plastic ground cloth, and I was out like a light.

A little later, we were awakened by the sound of helicopter machine gun fire.

"Those poor *compas* out there," said Esmeralda.

I didn't respond, but I could feel the knot in my throat now. It was 4 A.M. After a while, the helicopters left, so we went back to sleep. But soon I heard,

"Get up, *compas*! . . . psstt, get up!"

We collected our things quietly, quickly fell in, and left. Amazingly, we reached a lovely, big adobe house, where the owner gave us permission to cook and fix up a makeshift ward for any wounded that might come in. We set up an OR in an empty room, complete with operating and instrument tables, just in case.

The cooks made hundreds of tortillas and chicken soup. We were all so nervous. There was nothing to do but wait. How would the battle go? Would *compas* die? Would they take the position?

To calm ourselves and kill time, four of us got the owner's permission to cut cane in his field. We greedily sucked on one stalk after another—it was so sweet.

"Be careful! Look out for the spotter plane."

"Peel this for me, Chema. Thanks." I got covered in cane juice up to my elbows, without forgetting to keep a watchful eye on the plane.

The *compas* got back at sundown. Our battalion had only been the containment force and didn't suffer any casualties. The big news was that the *compas* had captured a 120mm mortar cannon. That was fabulous! They told us that the other battalion had gotten into the center of the town, but they had to withdraw when the helicopters came and the planes started bombing heavily.

It seemed to us that another incursion would be inevitable in retaliation for the captured cannon. The enemy was like a mad dog. The offensive indeed came, so we took off in *guinda*. We managed to outsmart them; they didn't detect us as we moved out, with branches tied to our backs as camouflage. We then set up ambushes in different places. But, unfortunately, a detachment of enemy soldiers happened upon a group of civilians in hiding, mostly women, children, and elderly people, and they killed every last one of them to make them pay for the lost cannon. There were sixty-six people massacred in all. That's how it is with the brave Atlacatl Battalion.*

Another day they discovered us. Bombs and mortars everywhere. We lay on our backs so we could see where the bombs were falling. One of the *compas* told me: "If you see a bomb coming at you, get up, run, and then hit the ground again—fast!"

After things calmed down, we were delighted when we came upon some cassava fields—we hadn't eaten for four days. We ate cassava until we got "cassavaed-out." We got bloated on cassava. That afternoon, when we started walking again, some of the *compas* were vomiting cassava, while others had cassava diarrhea. Cassava is great food, but after several days of not eating, it proved disastrous for our column.

A week later, Clodomiro, a *compa* from logistics, came over to me. "I'm going to Tenancingo to look for some books. Want to come?"

"Books? Around here?"

"Well, sure. There's got to be some since there was a library."

We headed off, along with César, another logistics *compa*. It was a beautiful sunny afternoon.

"There's a song by Carlos Mejía Godoy about Clodomiro, isn't there?"

"Yeah. The *compas* are always teasing me about it."

"Well, I like it."

After passing some coffee fields and a tobacco-drying shed, we reached the first houses. Tenancingo had been brutal-

---

*A U.S.-trained elite battalion of the Salvadoran army. It is reported to be one of the most aggressive and destructive of governmental troops.

ly destroyed in an air raid after the guerrillas attacked the army post there and had been the site of one of the most wanton civilian massacres in the war.

There were still fruit-bearing orange and almond trees in the yards. Clodomiro didn't take his eyes off me as he savored his orange. He told me he was going to take me to a lovely spot.

"You really know this place, don't you?"

"I was here when we took the post, and I've been back several times. I'll show you where the bastards were."

César had been noisily rummaging around in the rubble. Who knows what he was looking for. He looked out of place with his perfect teeth and his educated manner, which reminded me of an English lord's.

Leaving César to his searching, I followed Clodomiro around that ghost town until we reached the pharmacy. Inside, absolutely everything was destroyed. The counter was still standing, but its glass top had been broken, as well as the boxes and jars of medicine scattered on the floor.

"No bombs fell here in the pharmacy, but after the attack, the enemy returned, sacking everything that hadn't been destroyed in the bombing. They later said to the media that the guerrillas did it. The government wanted the civilians to fear us when they returned to their town. But, after such a bold-faced, bloodthirsty air raid, who would ever believe such a thing?"

There were some palm trees in the square in front of the municipal building and the church, one of the few intact edifices in town. Clodomiro explained that the soldiers had fled their headquarters and hidden in the church. The officer in charge then ordered the planes to destroy the whole town, except the church. Radio Farabundo Martí made a recording of these orders and later broadcast them to denounce the massacre that resulted.

Behind the church, we found some papaya trees with fruit ready to fall, which we savored while staring at the desolate destruction. The town smelled of death; the roofs of the houses had caved in, leaving just the facades. Finally, we came to the school, a big modern building with lots of classrooms and school benches. One room had hundreds of books, some of them still on the shelves, though most of them scattered on the floor. We looked through them in silence.

I decided on several: one about the Yaqui Indians of Mexico; another by Claribel Alegría, the title of which I don't recall; and a few more to give away to the *compas* back at the camp. Clodomiro picked up one by Bartolomé de las Casas to give to me. How strange it was to see so many books in one place after so many years! But it was getting late. Happy with our findings, we left to join the "English lord," who was still rummaging cheerfully in the debris.

"What did you find?" Clodomiro asked him.

"Nothing."

We then contined walking together to the outskirts of the town. When we got to the tobacco-drying shed, we gathered some leaves and rolled them into homemade cigars. As we walked on, the afternoon colors took us out of the war for a few moments. The atmosphere encouraged us to reminisce.

Clodomiro talked about his mother and his family, his unfinished university career, the urban guerrillas, the first underground explosives workshops in the city, and life in the mountains in 1979. I found myself admiring this man, with his rugged features and gentle expression. When I asked him why he had been struggling all his life, he began to recite Roque Dalton's "Love Poem":*

> The ones who widened the Panama Canal
> (and were on the "silver roll" not the "gold roll"),
> those who repaired the Pacific fleet
> in California bases,
> the ones who rotted in the prisons of Guatemala,
> Mexico, Honduras, Nicaragua,
> for stealing, smuggling, swindling,
> for starving,
> those always suspected of everything
> ("Allow me to place him in your custody
> for suspicious loitering
> aggravated by the fact of being Salvadoran"),
> those who pack the bars and whorehouses
> in every port and capital

---

*Roque Dalton, *Poems*, trans. Richard Schaaf (Willimantic, CT.: Curbstone Press, 1983). Reprinted with permission from Curbstone Press.

("The Blue Grotto," "The G-String," "Happyland")
the sowers of corn deep in foreign forests,
the crime barons of the scandal sheets,
those nobody ever knows where they're from,
the best artisans in the world,
those who were riddled by bullets crossing the border,
those who died from malaria
or scorpion bites or swarming bees
in the hell of banana plantations,
those who got drunk and wept for the national anthem
under a Pacific cyclone or up north in the snow,
the spongers, beggars, pot-heads,
the stupid sons of whores,
those who were barely able to get back,
those with a little more luck,
the forever undocumented,
those who do anything, sell anything, eat anything,
the first ones to pull a knife,
the wretched most wretched of the earth,
my compatriots,
my brothers.

We walked on in silence, interrupted only by Clodomiro occasionally repeating the line about "those who do anything, sell anything, eat anything."

Once back at camp I immediately went to Esmeralda to show her the books.

"That's great! But, they'll weigh down your pack," she said with her usual realism.

"Well, we'll just have to read them before we move on."

And a few days later we left the camp to go on another mission. Tejutepeque, damn Tejute.... This time our experience was really hell.

A sick *compa* named Roberto, as big as his malaria was bad, had to be carried with us in a hammock. We took turns carrying his heavy pack weighted down with ammunition, in addition to lugging our own. The column moved slowly, stopping often, with dogs barking at our advance.

Soon helicopters appeared, firing machine gun volleys and Bengal flares. We hit the ground. Dust and bullets filled the night. The tracer bullets sailed red and bright out of the choppers, rat-tat-tat-tat. I hated my damn camouflage pants, which had faded so much they were like a white flag in the middle of the night. When finally the helicopters laid off, we continued walking, suffering from acute drowsiness.

It was dawn when we reached the outskirts of Tejute. We stopped to rest under a big tree, but before long we were being fired on by a .50 machine gun which was located on a small hill just south of us. Again the helicopters came, this time loaded with troops; Cessna A-37's dropped bombs all over the place.

"Well, you could say we're surrounded," a *compa* explained calmly. "The enemy's dug in on that hill and the helicopters are landing on the other. And here we are right in the middle."

As if we weren't in enough trouble, some wounded in hammocks were brought in, and in the middle of the commotion, the MSU chief ordered us to pick them up and hit the road on the double. My heart was pounding in my mouth. I could practically chew it. It was, in fact, the only part of me that was marching double time because my legs simply felt paralyzed. I'd never seen such a godforsaken road as the one we had to run down. There wasn't a tree in sight to hide under. We were all mixed up together, combatants and support people. We quickly cut branches from a few bushes nearby to use as camouflage, while the planes nosedived on the other side of the town. We ran like hell but we didn't seem to get anywhere.

At last we reached a coffee field, where tall leafy shade trees offered some cover for a while. But then, directly ahead, we had to cross a pasture. Just as the first *compas* scrambled out of the coffee field into the open area, they were met by a heavy volley: rat-tat-tat-tat. Everyone hit the ground. Were they killed? Or waiting it out? I was soon relieved to see crawling butts and heads. But me? Go into that pasture?! No way! One of the cooks yelled something to me. Bullets were flying every which way and ricocheting off the trees. The coffee field, which had seemed so safe, was now a fucking shooting gallery; I took cover behind one big thick tree, but the bullets began ripping huge chunks right out of the trunk. It was as if some murdering enemy sniper had seen me and wouldn't stop. An eternity of feelings welled up in just fractions of a second. I made a run for it, zig-zagging just like we'd been instructed. It didn't even cross my mind that I still had Roberto's heavy pack, full of ammunition.

I ran a good distance, along with the cooks. At last we reached a cane field, but we were lost. We dragged ourselves along on all fours, passing under the nose of the biggest bull I've ever seen. Despite the shooting, the bull calmly kept on ruminating, watching us three little worms crawl in front of it. It made no threats of violence; it would have been just our luck if the bull were working for the *Guardia*, too! Then we had to go through a barbed wire fence. The cooks made it quickly, but I got caught since I hadn't removed my pack. Now the bull was coming towards me.

"*Compas!* I'm stuck!"

They came back and pried me loose. Once free, we all ran, convinced our lives depended on it.

We were cutting across a yard when we saw a peasant *shelling corn!* It was shocking to see this man working so peacefully, with bombs and bullets thundering around him. Crick, crack, crick. . . . He glanced at us and went right on shelling. I looked back several times just to make sure I wasn't hallucinating. His hands kept moving, he wasn't a ghost.

"Excuse me . . . could you please tell us where this road leads?"

"Well, to the right, to the center of Tejute, to the left, to Cojute."

"There's no other way to go?"

"Nope, that's it."

With great information like that, we made one clear decision—not to head for Tejute. We ran to the left. Suddenly, we saw men in green uniforms. It was some *compas!* They made a sign for us to come quickly.

Let's just say that I was always glad to meet up with the *compas*, but this time my feelings were simply imcomparable. They were a detachment from the other battalion on this front. There was their chief, blue-eyed Silvio, and Walter, the supply master. We withdrew in an orderly fashion, and despite bullets flying by and dust and dirt, we felt a lot safer.

We hid in small underbrush on a hill with our wounded, aware of our empty bellies. Walter squatted next to me. He was the only survivor of the massacre of the four Dutch journalists in 1981. He told me about when he went to Holland to testify about the killing. He had been received by the queen and didn't know much about protocol. Since he had seen the Dutch women kissing everybody, he thought that when he met the queen, it would be bad manners not to kiss her, too. So, just like that, smack, smack, he gave her a kiss on each cheek.

We felt our hunger once more. Walter had left his knapsack with strategic corn flour and sugar reserves back at camp since he was sure that we would have already taken Tejute and had a feast. I checked my pack, but all I could find was a plastic bag that had once contained sugar. Eagerly, we licked the few grains trapped by the humidity. We also devoured ripe red coffee beans, which have a white pulp under the shell that's a bit sweet if you suck on it.

Silvio, meanwhile, sent some *compas* to survey the situation and find water to treat the wounded. We stayed hidden with his battalion nearly forty-eight hours before going back to our own.

In the weeks that followed, we made camp in a lot of places, carrying out different missions, until one day we started hearing rumors that we were going to Chalate, beloved Chalate, our rear guard. It was December and the dry season was beginning. We really looked forward to returning, especially since a lot of the *compas* were from there. Christmas was coming and many had been granted permission to visit their families. I was happy, too, because I liked Chalate a lot; actually, I loved Chalate and its people. I had worked there before, and I missed my friends.

Rowing like mad, we crossed the Cerrón Grande reservoir at night. The mosquitoes lavished their attention on us, just as before. At last, I once again set foot in Chalate! As I got out of the boat, I slipped in the mud and literally kissed the ground. But who cares. . . . We were in Chalate!

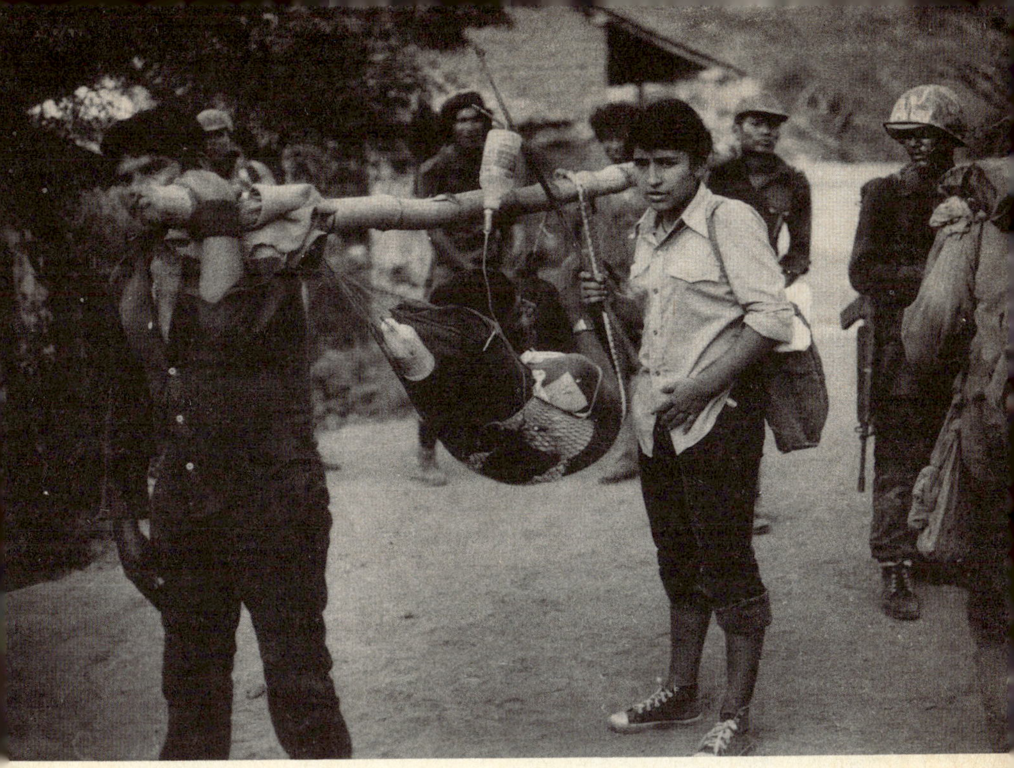

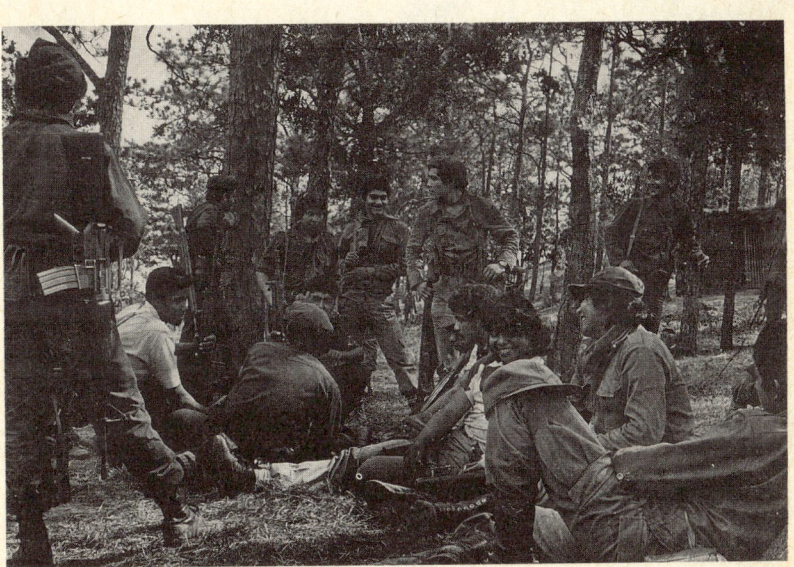

Top: The people's ambulance on the move. *Bottom:* Laughing and joking are a way of celebrating life.

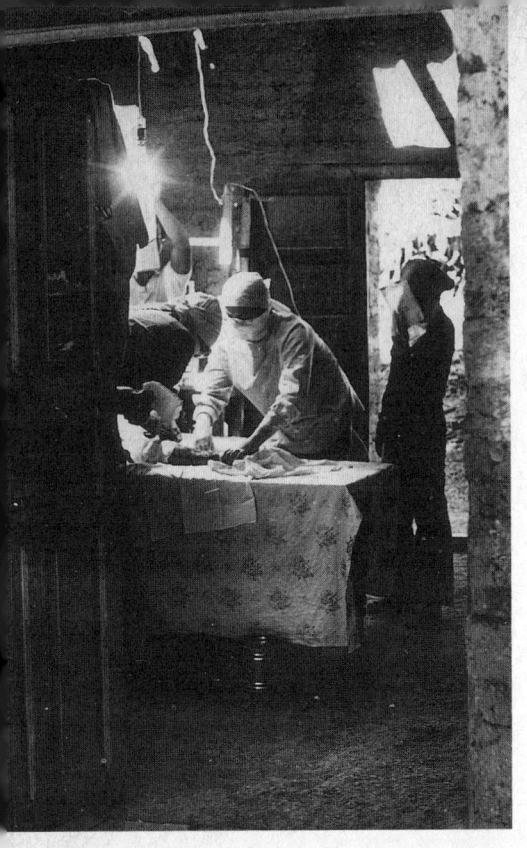

Top left: Who is more crucial: the one who holds the flashlight, the one who prepares the operating table, or the one who performs the surgery? *Bottom left:* When teeth ache, we have to pull them—there's nothing else we can do. *Bottom center:* In "B-52," the rehabilitation hospital, the wounded still make vital contributions. *Bottom right:* Toughen ourselves, yes, but never lose our tenderness. *Top right:* El Jicarito, August 1984: Air raids cause suffering and death, but they also strengthen our determination to work for a better society.

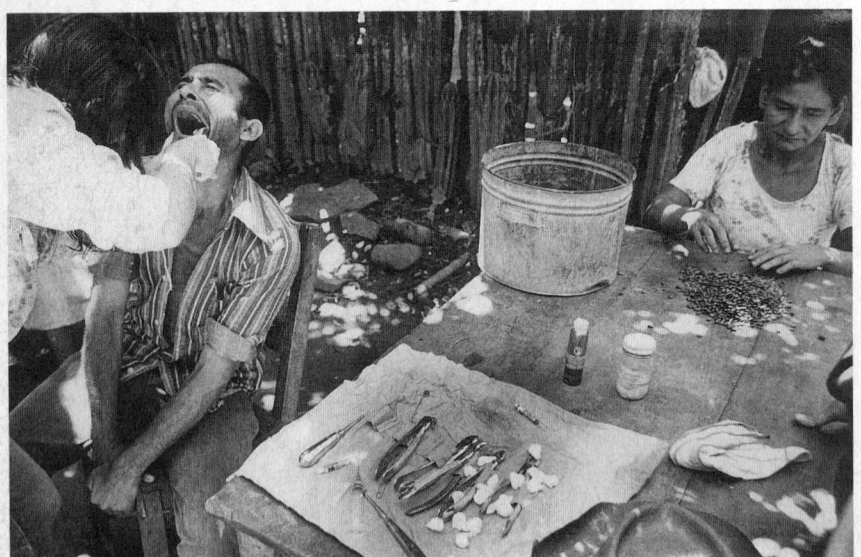
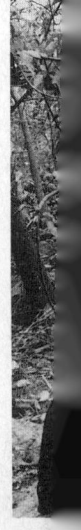

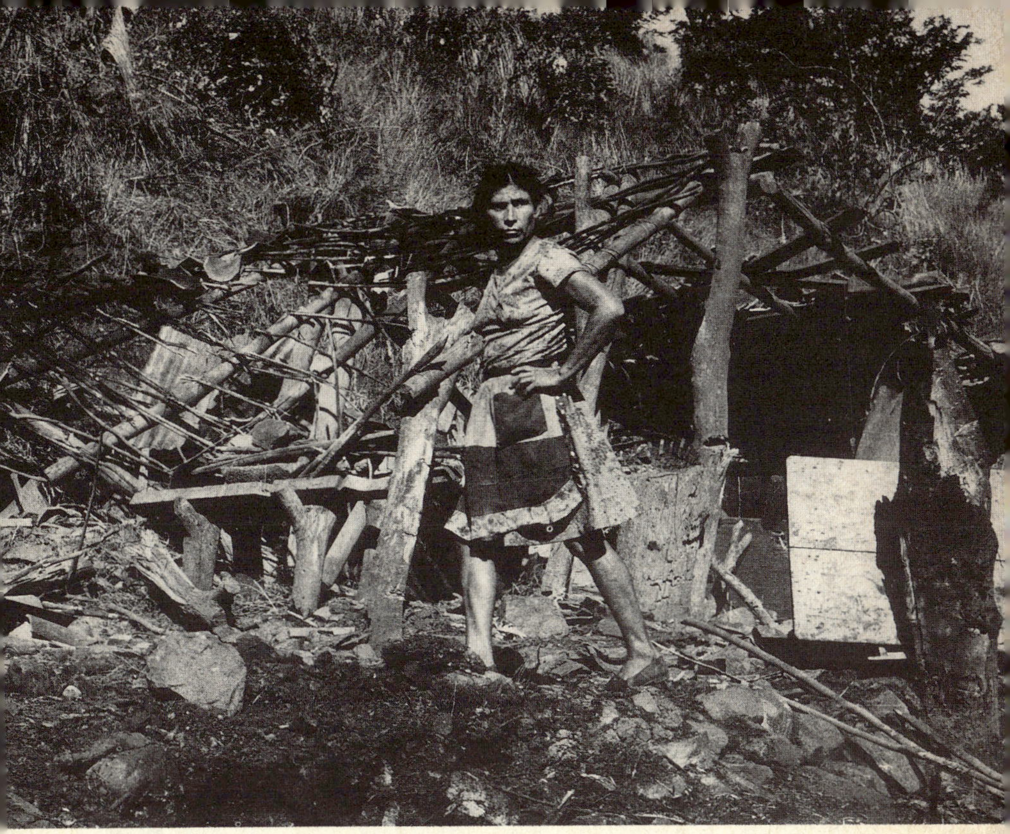

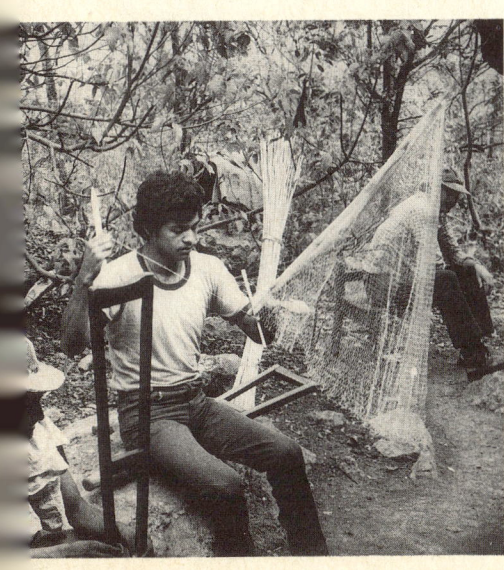
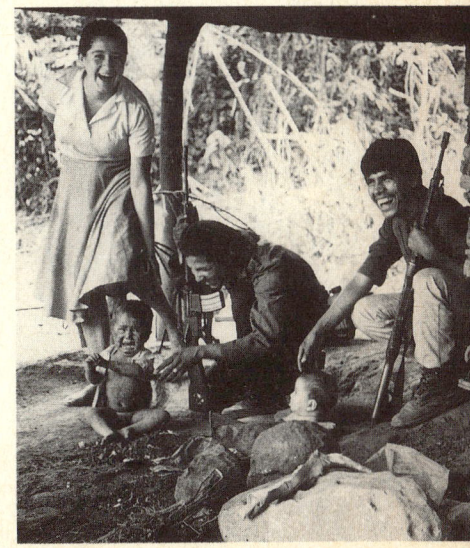

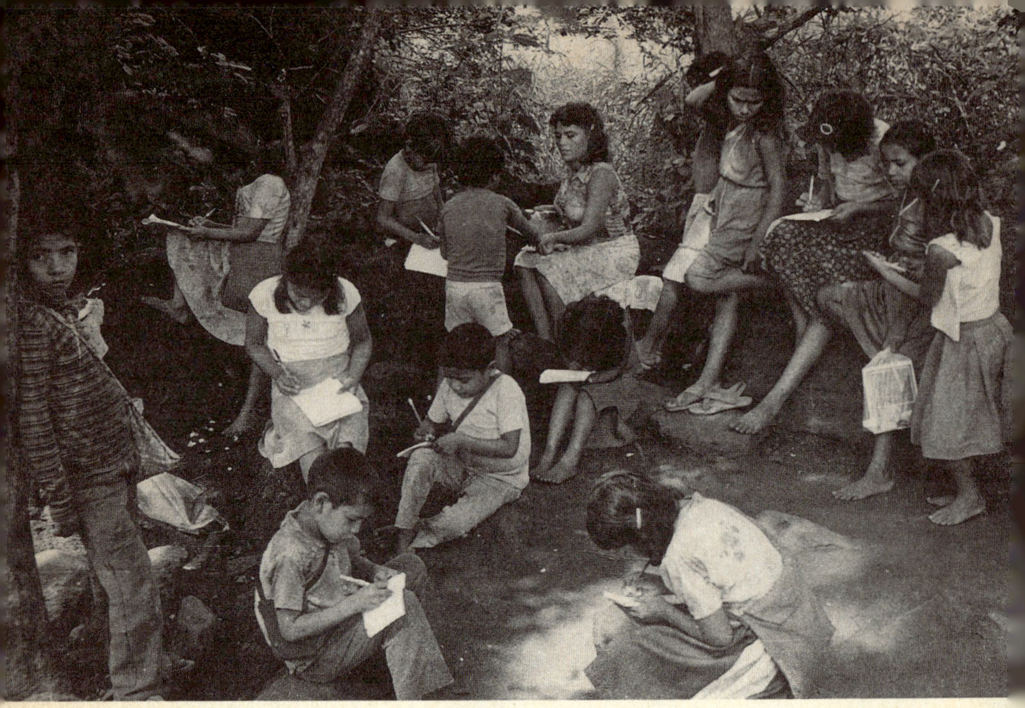

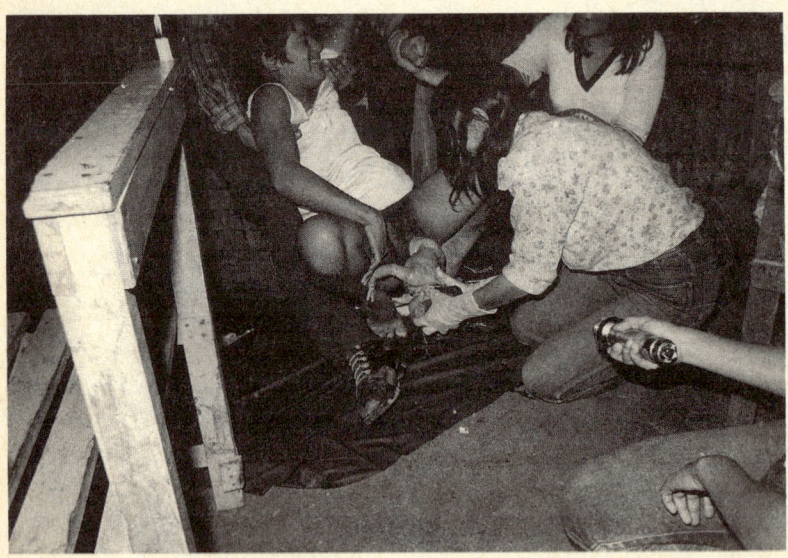

Top: Discovering, learning, and developing, so that they can come to have a say in their future. *Bottom:* Twenty minutes after an air raid, Julia, the head of the hospital, calls to Simón and Jezabel, the doctor: "Help me, the baby's coming!"

There's No More Medicine

"I called you in because the situation is serious," said Marilí, the chief of health care logistics. "I wanted you to know so that you can take whatever steps are necessary. All the medical logistics routes have been cut off. There's no telling for how long, but it would be advisable to think in terms of three, four, and even up to six months. We can't reorganize a strategic network like the one we had overnight, you know."

"Shit! What are we going to do?"

"I don't know exactly. We'll see. We've gotten out of more than one jam in this war. For the time being, I've checked the supply list, and our situation isn't critical yet. But, we'll have to give priority to the hospital; that's where the most urgent needs are. We'll continue to stock the clinics with basics as long as reserves last."

I had started working in a new team barely a month earlier. Our goal was to develop the people's clinics so that they could effectively and efficiently resolve the basic health problems of the population. How were we going to get this job off the ground, now that we lacked the fundamental materials?

I went to speak with José. I told him how pessimistic I felt, but all he said was: "You'll come out all right. Wait and see. You've always found the answers before. Just keep using your creativity."

They always said the same thing when the going got rough—they didn't have any idea how to do things either!

My new team included an internationalist doctor, Blanca, who didn't see a way out, either. But Angela, a peasant woman and health representative on the Subregional Government

Council, didn't get flustered. She told us, sensibly, "It's gonna be a bitch, but we'll handle it, just like always. We'll turn to nature once again, looking for the plants that can cure us."

We decided to call a meeting of all the health workers in the subregion immediately. The news travelled like wildfire. Complaints started: "Why have a meeting if there's no medicine? I don't have any shoes to walk that far." But with more perseverance than hope, we met on the scheduled day, to brainstorm about possible solutions.

The first goal was to tally the functions that the health workers could perform in the villages and hamlets. To our great surprise, most of them understood that in addition to healing duties, their task could involve preventive medicine as well as sanitary education. But what remained to be done, and what would be the most difficult, was finding a way to make the people understand the value of health care services that weren't strictly related to treatment.

We proposed taking monthly house-to-house surveys, dealing with the most common problems. This would allow us to get to know people well and help us understand their ideas and prejudices about health. After the first rains, gastroenteritis is always on the rise; we already knew that from experience. We could take advantage of this knowledge to interview people on the problem of diarrhea, which would then also allow us to broach the subject of building latrines. When planting season came around, on the other hand, we would research ways of improving our diet.

The proposal seemed realistic, but wasn't enthusiastically received. The younger, shyer health workers felt insecure about contacting and conversing with people this way. However, after a long discussion, the idea was accepted. We scheduled an evaluation of the results in a month's time.

At the same meeting, we proposed that we rely on natural remedies to heal people's ailments. A lot of people, including the health workers themselves, belittled medicinal plants. What to do? We decided to broaden the discussion, suggesting that natural medicines weren't just a strategic weapon against the enemy's siege, but also against dependence on multinational companies once the country was liberated. The idea was appealing. A few dared to support this approach, pointing out that plants are used to make some pills and that certain industrial pharmaceuticals have toxic effects.

With all this in mind, we drew up a list of the most useful herbs. As we did this we began to realize just how limited the *compas'* experience in this field was. Elizabeth and Angela were the most knowledgeable. However, in many cases they didn't agree on the utility of a particular plant, nor on the dose or length of treatment.

We decided, in any event, to keep a record of the herbal treatments we administered, in order to verify the efficacy of each natural remedy more scientifically. In this way we would begin to salvage this aspect of popular culture, and the results could later be disclosed to the other fronts. By the time we adjourned the meeting, our pessimism had disappeared and we even dreamed of making important advances in guerrilla medicine.

During the following weeks, our work with the population prompted us to concentrate our efforts on preventive measures and to tackle the problem of improving the people's diet. Since there were no large-scale invasions in 1983 and the first half of 1984, basic grain consumption had increased. Although vitamin and mineral requirements were supplied to some extent by vegetables and wild fruits, proteins were still severely lacking.

We suggested creating chicken farms in each locality. We proposed a budget for a model farm, selecting the location, and even found an old-timer who, right then and there, promised to raise the hens. With the local PPL committee, we made optimistic plans to give children, pregnant women, and elderly people one egg every other day. But no sooner had the government council approved the plan than the enemy changed its strategy, and we were forced out on *guindas* every four to eight weeks. There was nothing else to do but laugh at our own proposal. Nonetheless, we never completely abandoned the idea. When I left the Front, the *compas* were considering readapting it to the new situation.

Some of our other ideas were more within reach. Aided by

our surveys, we discovered that crops that were no longer seen in the zone, like sesame seed and peanuts, had been produced before the war. Both were valuable for their important fat allowances and modest vitamin and protein content. Furthermore, they could be sold in the outlying towns that traded with Chalatenango and San Salvador. The money would allow the people to purchase products that we couldn't produce. There was an added advantage: semame seeds could be suitable for mixing with our strategic reserve of flour and sugar, so vital for survival on the *guindas*. In time, thanks to our urging, several villages started growing these crops successfully.

It was Angela's job to help secure seeds with the help of the Subregional Government Council's production representative. She also trekked around the subregion publicizing our proposals, detecting problems, and helping to find ways to ensure successful harvests. However, Angela's promotion of good nutrition didn't stop there. She advised the *compas* on the benefits of planting fruit trees around their houses; in addition to nutritional benefits, the foliage would provide protection against aerial detection. She explained the value of garden vegetables, and other plants which they had traditionally grown. *Ayote*, a pumpkin-like squash, could also be grown over the roofing tiles so as to disguise them. To their surprise, people came to realize that radish greens could also be eaten. Little by little, all these proposals were put into practice.

During all this time, however, we were unable to solve the problem of the lack of pharmaceuticals. The basics that Marilí had promised us ran out in two month's time. In El Jicarito, an outspoken *compa* named Yanira came to see me after suffering from a headache for several days. When I recommended an herbal tea, she got angry. "I'm sure you have some pills for the other folks, but for a poor woman like me, you don't have shit!" she shouted and stalked away.

When someone came in with amoebic dysentery, I recommended a lemon juice cure first of all.

"But, there aren't any lemons, *compa*."

"Yes, there are. The trees in Llano Verde are full, and they're ripening right now."

"Well, maybe. But it's pretty far. Don't you have any pills, *compa?*"

"No, really, there aren't any. But you can make yourself a very effective brew with the bark from a mix of mango, avocado, *jiote colorado, copinol,* cashew, and sapota trees. Or just try sapota seed tea."

"Yeah, I know. The health worker already recommended that to me. I took it for two days and it didn't do anything for me."

"Of course, in two days the pills won't make you better either. It takes at least four or five days for itto start working and about ten until you feel OK again."

Other people rejected the infusions simply because they were bitter, looked unappetizing, or had a slimy consistency. It was so difficult. However, on the positive side, the consultations turned into occasions to chat about the efficacy of plants or about the situation we were going through. And with luck, the patients themselves ended up proposing previously unknown remedies.

While making home visits, I realized that a lot of people were in fact sick but no longer came to the clinic. They always said the same thing: "Well, it's no use, since there isn't even any medicine." We simply weren't getting through.

At monthly meetings, the health workers were disheartened and complained that people didn't pay attention to them, and sometimes even treated them badly, accusing them of favoritism. Several no longer received their basic grain subsidies from the population "since the clinic no longer does anything." It was difficult for these young women to influence their parents, aunts, uncles, and neighbors when they themselves had only just begun to assimilate new ideas. And besides, for the most part, they were shy young girls who lacked self-confidence.

So we found that the population resisted trusting the health workers and was hesitant to go to a clinic where all that was offered were natural remedies. As a result, attendance rose sharply at the hospital outpatient clinic, where there was still some medicine left, and a doctor.

From the point of view of their immediate needs, this reaction was understandable. But as part of the effort to organize a popular health care system with well-trained health workers in the middle of a people's war, it was a step backward. We didn't want to base health care around a few professionals and relatively sophisticated structures, which would unavoidably be inaccessible to the majority. Rather, we wanted to build a system which would at once respond to the population's most fundamental needs and increase the people's own self-confidence. Logically, the local clinic was the foundation of this project, and the village health worker, the instrument for carrying it out.

Even before this period of penury, we had tried to have the hospital favor the growth of the clinics, instead of curbing it. Our method was to have everyone first be examined in the clinic. If the health worker considered it necessary, she would give the patient a pass for the hospital. In it she noted her diagnosis and any treatment already provided. At the hospital, the doctor was expected to demand these references and reply to the health worker, assessing her diagnosis and mentioning the determining symptoms and the prescribed treatment. In this way, we had hoped to reinforce the people's clinic, develop health workers, and solve some of the population's health problems. We had already had problems with people's resistance to this idea and with a lack of cooperation on the part of some doctors, but when the clinic had nothing more than natural remedies to offer, our plan collapsed altogether.

What was behind this strong rejection of natural medicine? That was the basic question we found so hard to answer. Angela told me, "Don't let it get you down, man, these people are bull-headed. They tell me that what we say sounds great, but it isn't what they want. Our people struggle for the right to health care, but for them, this means modern medicine."

One day during a monthly meeting, one of the health workers told us a story that made me realize what Angela meant. The girl had had an argument with a *compa* because she had refused the woman a packet of oral rehydration salts. Just because it was called "oral serum," people attributed it with extraordinary powers, far beyond its usefulness for diarrhea. People's faith in "serum" is understandable when one knows that before the war, unscrupulous health workers charged up to fourteen colones to administer "serum," that is, IV saline solution, billing it as "nutrition against weakness."

Domenica, Angela's mother, helped us understand the situation better. A strong woman, already over seventy, she had raised nine children by growing garden vegetables, baking bread, and selling what wild fruit she could glean in the woods. Domenica indeed knew about herbal medicine. When she happened upon an herb or tree that she recognized for its healing properties, she took it home and planted it. Her medicinal garden helped her over the hard times.

I asked her why the people had lost their faith in plants and herbs.

"Years ago, there just wasn't anything else. In my case I learned everything I could because I had no choice; it was the only way I could raise my kids. I couldn't even afford the colón they charged at the Health Center in Arcatao. There were days when that was all I earned. But later, when they started selling pills in the street, folks were thrilled, even though people went without eating in order to pay for them. Everyone was talking about them. Even on the radio they repeatedly told us how great those drugs were. And so, little by little, people just left the plants to the old-timers. That was their mistake, if you ask me. Look at me, I've never been to a doctor in my life!"

Indeed, few people went to her for advice, despite her obvious experience. Nor, unfortunately, did she worry about systematically transmitting her store of knowledge to her children.

Suddenly, the reason for the rejection of herbal medicine seemed obvious. In modern times, plants were nothing more than a poor person's resource, not an alternative, consciously chosen for its healing value, and much less out of any desire to preserve these aspects of popular culture. Herbs responded to nothing more than the tyranny of need. Thus the prevalence of poverty had distorted concepts about medicine. This was indeed a negative starting point for building a truly revolutionary health care system.

For too long, we had taken for granted the ideal image of a people struggling for their liberation. We were encouraged by the stories of the liberated zones of Vietnam, Guinea Bissau, and Algeria. We had thought that an indigenous peasant people, living close to nature, would have a true working knowledge of medicinal plants. We thought that recovering their medicinal culture would fulfill a deep-seated need. Now we discovered that if we didn't take into account the destruction and distortion of that culture, we wouldn't get anywhere.

We were forced to look for a more realistic and attainable project, something amenable to both the people's vision of health care and our own. Angela met with the Government Council and reported the outcome. "There is a small fund that can be used to purchase medicines through some collaborators. It's not much money, but it will do until the clandestine routes can be reopened."

So we decided that restocking our clinics with medicines was the best course. Despite this apparent defeat, the experience had been fruitful. We learned a lot about plants. We could now teach industrial and herbal treatments concurrently. Health care work became more comprehensive. But above all, given the limitations of the past and the present, a great debate had been initiated, and we had already gone a good stretch in the long road to transformation.

The Right to Eat

In a country where people are often short of food, and even more so in a war zone, those who don't produce their own food are very vulnerable. Health workers don't have their own fields, yet in the people's war it is felt that they do work for the collective good, and thereby earn their right to receive food from the community. Getting the population to recognize the value of their work in the popular clinics and providing them with basic grains, salt, and sugar, plus notebooks and shoes, was one of our team's main problems.

Some PPL committees saw to the health workers' needs punctually; others complied with their responsibility, but did so irregularly; and a minority delayed giving provisions for months on end. For a while, Los Amates was the most negligent committee of all.

Ironically, to us this village was synonymous with abundance. Located at the concourse of the Sumpul and Guancora Rivers, its fertile riverbanks yielded two abundant corn crops per year. There was a Production Brigade located there, which, along with raising vegetables and fruit, had dairy cows and ran a fishing cooperative. When the Sumpul reservoir was low, people could be seen catching fish by hand that had been left stranded in the shallow pools.

For the past two years, Eva had been Los Amates' health worker. She had accumulated a considerable experience in medicine, first at a guerrilla base camp, and later by working in the villages for four years. At forty, she was fascinated by health care, which she considered a concrete way of breaking out of her traditional role as a woman and peasant, with no future other than housework. At night, she melted down leftover candle stubs in order to make a new taper and study *Where There*

Is No Doctor in its light. Since her knowledge of medicine was greater than that of the rest of my workshop participants, I gave her private classes. She came to see her work more comprehensively; she generally followed up on patients and didn't limit herself to prescribing drugs but tackled problems of hygiene and prevention as well, giving talks to the women from the women's organization (AMES) and broaching these subjects at village assemblies.

However, Eva had a difficult personality and her way of handling others left a lot to be desired. She could be really disagreeable sometimes and readily scolded patients who didn't follow her instructions. If people insisted on a pill or a shot that she didn't deem necessary, they got a good tongue-lashing. Although this wasn't reason enough to deny her provisions, it was used as a pretext by some PPL representatives.

Eva was overwhelmed by all her responsibilities: health work, household tasks, efforts to obtain food. She was really bad at organizing her time. She would start to make tortillas and then suddenly shift her attention to write something down or rearrange medicine bottles, burning the tortillas in the meantime.

Among civilians, it was quite unusual for a woman to live apart from her relatives as Eva was doing. As a result, loneliness weighed enormously on her. Her only company at the clinic was Don Jacobo, a niggardly old grouch who expected her to wait on him like a spouse or maid in exchange for housing the health center in his private home. Eva absolutely refused to submit and the two lived in a permanent state of cold war.

Like the rest of the health workers, Eva needed things that were difficult for the popular government's budget to provide. For example, even though Salvadoran peasants have always gone barefoot, the health workers needed shoes for long hikes to fetch medicines or attend meetings. In the war, shoes are strategically important for everyone, but unfortunately, even the cheapest are expensive. There was just too little money to go around.

In each hamlet, the individuals who were not organized in a Production Brigade—where work is purely collective—

devoted a few work days each week for the benefit of the community, or more precisely, for the widows, volunteer peasant teachers, and health workers. While the collective harvest lasted, there weren't any major problems; however, this was not the case when it ran out towards the end of the productive cycle.

In addition to this harvest, the PPL had other resources. Goods were sold in the people's store at a ten percent profit margin. These earnings were earmarked, on one hand, to augment the shop's tiny capital and, on the other, to finance social projects. Nevertheless, when it came time to assign the profits, some committees gave priority to the store, disregarding the teachers' and health workers' needs. The widows, by contrast, were generally taken care of. Los Amates was one of these hamlets, leaving Eva no alternative but to look for leaves and fruits in the hills, garden the AMES vegetable plot, and even fish the Sumpul with her friend Mirna, an activity in which women rarely engaged. She also baked and sold *salporas*—little cakes made from corn or sorghum flour.

All these efforts to obtain food increased Eva's feelings of resentment and frustration, since they took time away from her real duties. She was extremely thin, partly because of her highstrung nature, and became even more so as she was obliged to endure severe shortages for weeks at a time.

Most people were conscious of her situation. Now and then somebody sent her fish or fruit; others invited her to eat with them, but she almost always refused. On several occasions, I tried to reason with her, but she refuted my arguments. "I don't want their pity. I want my own food to fix as I like."

In reality, the problem was the PPL's responsibility. So I met with old Justo, the representative in charge of health, but my efforts got me nowhere. The old guy was too weak-willed for the job. After every meeting, he went home convinced he had done a good job, even though he never managed to impress on the president of the local committee the importance of health work. People realized he lacked dynamism, and fortunately, didn't vote for him in the next election. But for now, Eva's problem remained.

The person in control of finances was Ulises, the president. He was more educated than most and had had the chance to travel to other countries. In addition to talking a good line, he had another characteristic: he didn't always keep his promises. I insisted on the importance of delivering Eva's food allocations regularly. But the situation went from bad to worse because he didn't respect the agreements we had reached. And it came to a crisis during the final weeks of scarcity at the end of the production cycle. Eva was practically not eating at all. So once more, I went to find Ulises.

"It's just that there's no grain left," he replied.

"OK. Here there's not, but there's still some to be had on the Front."

"Look, Eva doesn't have any family and she can go out looking for herself. Right now my job is to get grain for the Brigade."

"When you get some, give Eva a little. She's already spent a lot of time scavenging."

"Perhaps, but the money that the Council gave me is only for the Brigade."

"OK. But Eva works for the Brigade, too. She does her best to keep them as healthy as possible."

"But with that money, I can't do anything for her."

"Then use money from the store."

"But there's no grain to buy. We're using a special connection to get some for the Brigade."

"Well, give her the money and I'm sure she'll find some to buy. That's what they're doing in El Tamarindo."

"Maybe. But tomorrow the shopkeeper's going to town to buy supplies and we can't spare any cash."

"OK, then as president, you can borrow some sorghum from Don Jacobo. I know he still has enough."

"No, the old guy won't sell. Excuse me, I've got a meeting," he said nervously, and left without letting me say anything else.

It was unfortunately all too clear to me that Ulises lacked both the will and the vision necessary to solve Eva's problem. Upon returning to the clinic, I let off so much steam about

Ulises' behavior that Don Jacobo ended up giving Eva some sorghum. But this didn't take care of the root of the matter.

In our next work session, Angela, Blanca, and I talked it over. I favored asking the Council to take severe measures with committees that didn't respect their obligations to the health workers and, more specifically, I wanted them to sanction Ulises. Blanca and Angela disagreed. Both felt the way to solve the problem was to take it to the people. Finally, we decided to demand that an assembly be held to deal with the matter.

Right after that meeting, I ran into María, an important party representative in the subregion.

"I know that guy's no good," she responded. "But what can we do? He had prestige with the people and they voted for him. All we can do now is wait for the next elections. I think the folks here have also seen that he's inept. That's how we all learn, and that's what this is all about."

During my next visit to Los Amates, I talked to several well-respected members of the community: Leonel, the militia chief; Mauricio, the former head of the Production Brigade and ex-member of the PPL; and Mirna. They all agreed that calling an assembly was the best way out.

"But don't attack Ulises directly," Mauricio advised me, "because if he thinks you want the assembly for that, he won't call it properly, and almost no one will show up. He's always saying that people don't help Eva because she's so irritable. So suggest an assembly to deal with the problem between Eva and the others."

A few days later all the villagers, as well as Angela and I, gathered under a big banyan tree next to the PPL house. Angela spoke on our and the Council's behalf, then Leonel reported on the military situation. Finally Ulises brought up the "problem of the clinic."

At first, the assembly maintained a cautious silence. But then, Eva asked to speak. "Friends, I know you have several complaints about my work, so please speak up. We all need criticism in order to change and I'm ready to take it into account."

With that, several people decided to talk. Some complained that when they went to the clinic for a consultation, they didn't find Eva.

"It's because I'm out looking for firewood. That's why I posted a schedule."

"But that schedule business doesn't seem right to me. When I'm in the neighborhood, I want to make the most of it, without having to wait."

Several times, people's criticisms of her treatments obliged me to intervene to endorse her skills as a health worker and explain that her work was subject to my supervision and control. When these subjects had been sufficiently discussed, Mauricio tactfully went to the point: Eva was not getting the support she merited. With this, a silence fell on the meeting and it was a good while before anyone dared break it.

"We don't like it when Eva rejects what we offer her. But that's how she is. What can we do? So now she shouldn't complain," said one of the women.

Mirna asked for the floor.

"The *compa's* right, that's how Eva is and we all know it, but we are offended anyway. Not only that, people see her selling *salporas* and some think maybe she doesn't need support any more. What's more, perhaps on account of her vice, many figure that she doesn't consider food important. I, for one, know that she needs help, but others don't see it like that."

These comments confused me. I didn't know if Mirna was criticizing Eva or the villagers. Indeed, Eva was fond of tobacco. At night, she often rolled herself a little stogie, using a notebook page or other equally inappropriate paper.

Mauricio spoke again. "It's true that Eva likes to smoke and not all women are accustomed to that, but that's not the problem. Although she may be proud and speak gruffly, we mustn't forget that she's a damn good health worker. Paco says so himself. She's doing a good job for us and we're obliged to support her. In this respect, I must confess that sometimes I have a little something—fish or avocados—and I don't always think of her, even though I should. But, as far as basics go, it's the PPL's responsibility. Our community resources are certainly scarce, but I think we'd all agree, there's enough for a few tortillas."

People backed him up. Ulises stood up and began talking non-stop. He went on and on about all the efforts he was making for the people, until finally, he declared, "I know that the *compa* works hard and is sacrificing a lot for us, and it's true that there have been times when we've been unable to provide for her. But I now promise to meet our obligation to her, whenever it's possible."

This "whenever it's possible" worried me, but at least he'd been somewhat self-critical.

"I feel really good about this assembly," said Leonel standing up. His speech was a perfect summing up of revolutionary practice. "Solving problems like this is a concrete way of advancing towards a society of new men and women. We've seen the humility of those who criticize and of those who accept criticism. We hope that Eva will mend her ways and that the committee will take its responsibility towards her more seriously. I think we're lucky to have someone like her who is so dedicated to helping and teaching us."

In the following weeks, Eva's situation indeed improved, though it still left something to be desired. New committee elections were soon held, and luckily, Mirna was voted in instead of Ulises.

"We'll calculate better what we have in the collective supplies so that it lasts us longer and Eva gets taken care of," Mirna explained to me on my first visit to her as president. "That way the profits from the store will be principally used for restocking."

And with a frank smile, she added, "In any case, I sure don't want to have you and Angela on my back!"

A Shark Attacks Our Workshop

"Paco, did you see the plane?" Miriam, the health worker from Los Planes, anxiously asked me as I entered her house, one midday in early August of 1984.

"Yeah, of course. It flew right over my head."

"I wonder what the hell it was up to? It only made one pass and was gone. That's weird."

"Who knows. Perhaps it was an exercise; they probably call it 'practice in enemy territory.'"

Everybody in Los Planes was very upset about the low-flying enemy bomber. It didn't actually pass directly over the hamlet, but it came close enough to cause real concern. The people there had considerable past experience with air raids. Some six feet from Miriam's house, there was a big hole where a 500 pound bomb had fallen a little less than a year before. Although that one didn't explode, and militiamen had later dug it up in order to retrieve the explosive material, seven other bombs had maimed and killed several villagers during that same attack. Despite general nervousness, Miriam and I had a good talk that afternoon about her work.

I completed my visit and started back to El Jicarito where, for the past several weeks, I had been giving a workshop to the health workers from Los Planes and other nearby villages. The path twisted its way up a steep slope planted with sweet, young corn that showed promise of a good harvest. After El Jicarito had been destroyed during a government army offensive in November 1982, the population had returned and rebuilt it. They made their new homes, really nothing more than shacks, from wooden planks and scraps of zinc found in San Isidro and other abandoned towns. Experience had taught them to dig air raid shelters and trenches before considering their job done.

Early the next morning, Miriam and the other health workers installed themselves around a wobbly table in El Jicarito's popular clinic, ready for the workshop to begin.

"Let's review a bit. What did we talk about last week?" I started.

Embarrassed laughter.

"About 'that time of the month,' " Lilian, a fifteen-year-old health worker from a neighboring hamlet, finally ventured.

"How do we say that in medical terms?"

"The . . . period."

"Is there another word?"

"Menstration," Lilian responded a bit hesitantly.

"Okay, almost. Men-stru-ation," I spelled out. "Why do women have it?" I asked the others.

"Isn't it because the little egg didn't stick?" Luz, another teenage health worker, suggested.

"That's right. But where is it that it didn't stick?"

"In that thin skin, the one you said was so soft," answered Narcisa, one of the girls in charge of El Jicarito's clinic.

The review was going well; it was clear that last week they had been interested and had paid better attention in class than usual. At this point, Lidia, nine months pregnant and suffering from severe anemia, walked by, which gave me a perfect opening to discuss her disease and its repercussions on the fetus.

We had barely begun when suddenly there was a loud noise.

"The plane!" Miriam shouted, horror stricken. "The damn thing's getting ready to attack us here!"

She was still screaming as everyone jumped up. Glancing at the sky, in a fraction of a second, I saw a plane taking position to attack. I raced with the others, trying to make it to the trench about thirty feet away. We didn't even get halfway there when we heard the plane dive overhead, ready to drop the first bomb.

"Hit the ground!" someone shouted.

We threw ourselves down. For several devastating moments, all we heard was the terrorizing buzz of the diving plane and then, an explosion thundered inside each of us and, at the same time, a few feet away. The tall grass bent over us; a blast of air lacerated the long flexible leaves of nearby banana plants. In seconds, the plane pulled up to a higher altitude, roaring mercilessly. Reduced to nothing more than fear and the desire to survive, we seized the chance to make a run for the trench. At the instant in which I reached it and threw my body down, the earth shook with a tremendous roar.

"Shit! That one fell really close!"

Again the shriek of the plane and a spasm in the bowels of the earth. Several rocks, embedded in the trench walls, loosened and fell in. Shrapnel buzzed, slicing the air and the plants, like a sadist with a thousand razor sharp switchblades seeking victims.

I thought, "I'll never get out of here alive," and wondered for an instant which of the doctors was on duty at the hospital: if I got hit in the abdomen. . . . The earth soon shook again and the shiny belly of the plane, like that of a ferocious shark, streaked overhead. From that moment on I thought of the plane as The Shark, as in Willie Colón's song.

I lay on my back, wracked with anxiety, surveying the narrow strip of blue sky that the trench allowed me to see. We were so cramped together that my head was lodged in between Lilian's legs. I was feeling neither shame nor embarrassment. Perhaps this proximity somewhat consoled us in the midst of our vulnerability. The murderous Shark blanked out the patch of blue sky and showed its paunch time and time again. Lilian pleaded loudly: "Deliver us from this evil spirit. . . . God, make this demon go away. . . . Protect us, Holy Father. . .. I beg you and the Holy Virgin, make this damn thing leave!"

It wasn't her faith that impressed me so much as the realization that, by having it, she had a tremendous resource against impotence. The Cessna A-37 continued to hurl terror, trying to crush out our fragile lives and hopes with its hideous power. But soon the noise started to move in another direction. Now the plane was focusing death on another part of the hamlet. That might have been a relief to me, but how could it be, knowing that it was now Narcisa's and Luz's parents, my friends, and my comrades who were the targets of this savage bombing?

Suddenly the image of the United States Congresspeople who approve funds for anti-guerrilla struggles in faraway lands flashed through my mind. It was shocking to know that they refused to recognize what they were really financing: the destruction of the lives of girls like Lilian, Miriam, and the others, who were doing nothing more than trying to learn something about health in order to improve conditions for themselves and their neighbors.

Once the plane finally departed, the echo of its horrible buzz and the image of the Shark's dreadful belly hung on in our memories. Prudently, we waited. Would the plane come back? How much time had gone by? Twenty minutes? An hour? I couldn't erase the vision of the Shark from my mind. Everything became a blur; I didn't even know if there had been one plane or several.

In the first instant after I carefully emerged from the trench, the hamlet looked intact. But upon taking a few steps toward it, I noticed that all the banana plants had their leaves slashed and looked as if a hurricane had whirled through them. Then I saw a thick branch of a sturdy *sicahuite* tree, completely shattered by shrapnel.

With each step, the evidence of destruction increased. A bomb had blown half the clinic's roof off; its beams and tiles were shattered to pieces. The zinc walls were twisted and ruined. Inside, there was nothing but debris. Of the three houses closest to where that bomb had fallen, not even a post was still standing; they were obliterated by the force of the shock wave and the shrapnel. But strangest of all, there was not a single sound to be heard—absolute silence reigned. Surely there were wounded, but where?

Thoroughly scared, fearing that the terrible beast would return, the health workers and I headed towards the center of the hamlet together. Some 200 yards from the clinic, I saw that my patient Yanira's house hadn't been too badly affected, but just beyond it, all that remained of what had been five houses was scattered debris, vestiges of chairs, tables, clay pots and water jugs, all in pieces. Still nobody. Only the pervading silence.

Hate, fear, and sadness overwhelmed me. Several of the health workers spoke to me, but I don't know what they said. Without paying any attention to them, I numbly walked on, discovering that more of the houses and gardens, which had been so familiar to me, had been destroyed. Suddenly I stumbled over something at the base of a *sicahuite* tree. It was Melida, still spread-eagled on the ground, in shock and fearing the plane's return. She spoke to me so excitedly that I couldn't understand her. Her skin was covered with countless red blotches; her face was full of suffering and anguish.

At last, she got up and was able to make me understand that in the large ditch at the other side of the ruins, which minutes before had been her house, there were some injured *compas*. I went over to see. A woman who looked about thirty years old and a little girl lay dead. Their bodies showed neither gashes nor wounds, but instead were grotesquely crumpled up from the force of the shock wave, like thin pieces of paper. I didn't recognize them. They had probably come from a nearby hamlet to sell custard apples, for next to their bodies, baskets and fruit were strewn on the ground.

Just then, I heard someone shouting my name. It was Jonson, the *compa* in charge of health in the local PPL committee. He was hurrying along a narrow path, carrying a child, about eight years old, in his arms.

"Over here, Paco, hurry! It's Reinita. She's real bad." The *compa's* voice neared hysteria. The girl was Jonson's granddaughter, and I knew how much he loved her.

At that same moment, another *compa* caught up with me, asking me to go see Lola, Leonardo, and Genaro's old sick mother.

"Her throat's slit, you'd better hurry."

The initial shock had passed. Now things happened rapidly. Miriam ran to see to Reinita and I rushed off to tend to old Lola.

The bomb had hit a huge banyan tree right outside the old woman's house. The tree, whose main branches had measured some five feet in diameter, was reduced to a bare trunk. Nearby, Leonardo's mother lay on the ground of her house, which had been simply blown away. Another elderly woman, who had been fortunate and managed to find protection by wedging herself between two huge boulders, told us that Lola had mustered the strength to get up from her sickbed, but the bomb had exploded before she could reach safety. She was over seventy years old. Leonardo, the son with whom she lived, hadn't been home during the bombing. Like most of the men, he had been out in the cornfield.

I examined her. A fragment had wounded the poor woman only superficially, but she was in shock, her lungs full of exudate on account of the damage from the shock wave. Barely conscious, she only groaned and stared straight ahead. I gave her an injection to relieve the pain.

"The injection will give her strength," Leonardo half stated, half asked.

"No, it'll just ease the pain."

His brother Genaro, the militia chief, arrived on the scene shortly after. Looking at his mother, he asked me, "How is she?"

I shook my head to tell him that there was no hope.

"We're going to gather the wounded at Orlando's house a little outside the village," he told me. Next, he turned to his brother and, after a moment's hesitation, said, "Leave her here, then."

He quickly withdrew in order to continue organizing the evacuation of the wounded. I was sure he had had to master his feelings. At that moment, he couldn't respond to his mother's situation alone, but had to act as the son of the whole people.

"We're not going to move her?" Leonardo asked sadly.

He was the bachelor son, the one who had carried her on his back in the *guindas* until he had found some safe place to hide her. His expression was neither dramatic nor tragic, just sad.

"No, *compa*. She's got very little time left. Stay with her. She's going to need you."

I then hurriedly left Lola to Leonardo's care. As I climbed the hill that took me to the center of the hamlet, my hatred and rage grew. The slopes were covered with *compas* evacuating wounded; scattered along the path, every so often, were the dead remains of chickens and roosters, the people's sole wealth. Behind Yanira's house, members of the militia were digging out a caved-in *tatu*.* I didn't stop. I wanted to get back to Miriam and the child, Reinita, as quickly as possible.

"What took you so long? She's dying on us. Miriam was at a loss what to do," Jonson said to me when I got there.

Leaving her in her grandfather's arms, I uncovered the girl so I could examine her. She was suffering intensely, but was still conscious and talking normally.

The skin and the first layer of muscle of almost her entire back, the entire lumbar region and most of the dorsum, had been blown away. The spinal column was exposed, visible from the sacrum to the shoulder blades, and miraculously intact. I could count each vertebra and see the white ligaments between them. What remained of the muscles was covered with dirt and bits of grass.

I was horrified, uncertain how to proceed. The bottles of sterilized water that we kept in the clinic to wash wounds had been smashed in the raid. Luz brought a big jug of drinking water. Aided by Jonson, his wife, and Luz, who held the girl down, Miriam and I proceeded to pour the water over the child's open back to clean off at least a little of the dirt. Then we wrapped her in clean rags, in order to send her to the hospital where they would do an adequate cleansing. The child wrestled and screamed, calling out for her mother and invoking help from God. Two militiamen arrived carrying a hammock slung on a bamboo pole to transfer her to Orlando's house, but I insisted that they take the child directly to the hospital. Luz accompanied her with more analgesic for the journey.

When I got to Orlando's house, the militiamen were preparing more hammocks, while the health workers were tending the wounded. All the villagers that could were partici-

---

*A concealed hole in the ground, used either as an air raid shelter or as a hiding place for food, medical supplies, arms, and other valuables. *Tatus* are also used for concealing wounded and disabled people, as well as children and the elderly, during *guindas*.

pating in one way or another. Some *compas* brought boiled water, while others found horses to transfer the less critical cases. Narcisa took care of her twelve-year-old brother, who had been hit in the Achilles' tendon by a piece of shrapnel while running to a trench. He had spent the whole air raid lying on the ground where he fell, his foot bleeding profusely.

There were others less seriously wounded: a four-year-old boy had been struck in the head but luckily didn't receive any cranial lesion. His father, who had just left the hospital after recovering from wounds suffered in another bombardment, was also bleeding.

"Twice now, God has granted me life!" he exclaimed.

Once the wounded were on their way to the hospital, I learned by talking with Orlando that I hadn't yet been aware of the magnitude of the tragedy. Reinita was the only survivor of a *tatu* where Lidia, her mother, three brothers and sisters, and two other *compas,* Ernesto and Lupe, had all died. It was Lidia who that very morning had prompted our discussion of anemia and its effects on the fetus. They had seen the plane coming and had run to a shelter, which proved too small for all of them. Ernesto remained half-exposed in the entrance, which undoubtedly had allowed the pilot to locate the group and target a direct hit. But, what accounted for wounds like Reinita's? The shock wave? The *tatu* caving in? Shrapnel?

Later, when I was back in the center of the hamlet, I took a closer look to try to figure out what had happened. There were practically no craters or big holes, which made me think that the enemy had not used conventional bombs, which explode on ground contact and plunge deep into the earth on impact. Shrapnel from those rebound upward to form a kind of upside down umbrella of flying metal, from which you can usually escape harm by just lying flat on the ground. No doubt, this time we had been subject to an attack by bombs "with a stick on the nose," as the *compas* describe them. These bombs have a contact bar in front, activating them at the slightest friction of matter against the bar, often before the bomb itself hits the earth, which explains why they leave no craters. When they do explode, the shrapnel rains all over the place and spreads out horizontally like an immense sea of red-hot metal, razing everything in its path. Furthermore, the shock wave of such a bomb has greater range and force; it is almost impossible to escape the impact, unless you are in a trench.

These treacherous devices are aseptically called anti-personnel bombs. It's rumored that one of the Yankee advisors in El Salvador is claiming his patent rights on it. True or not, it was overwhelming to see the effects of such genius placed at the service of death.

Some of the survivors started to rummage through the ruins of their dwellings, looking for anything salvageable. As poor as these people had been before, they were now reduced to pure misery.

Suddenly I heard Melida calling to me from a semi-destroyed house, where she and her family had taken refuge. I walked over to see how she was.

"The bombing wasn't enough for you, was it? You still had to trample me," she said laughingly recalling our encounter after the raid.

"What are those blotches on your skin?"

"Just think, I spent the whole attack behind that *sicahuite* tree. I didn't dare move an inch for fear that they would detect me. But the trunk was infested with ants and I had to put up with swarms of them biting me all over. When the bomb fell that killed that woman and the little girl, I got covered with dirt. I'm only alive thanks to God and that *sicahuite* tree."

Later, a little further up the hillside, the militiamen were repairing Yanira's slightly damaged house.

"We have to get it fixed up. A lot of people are going to sleep here," one of the *compas* explained.

The bodies of the victims—Lidia, her three children, Ernesto, Lola, and Lupe—lay on the porch of a semi-intact house nearby. A little to one side were the cadavers of the two fruit vendors. All of them were wrapped in patched blankets, and adorned with flowers and fresh cut boughs; two candles, which kept going out every couple of minutes from the breeze, were placed next to them by the villagers to honor them.

People arrived from neighboring hamlets. The men were

up on a nearby hilltop digging a communal grave; the women prayed and wept.

Their sobs grieved me but, at the same time, surprised me. Until then, I had only witnessed funerals in the hospital. There, the suffering was converted into political rage and subliminated. Discipline and self-control were ever present. What was the meaning of this openly emotional response to death?

"We don't cry over fallen guerrillas, we follow their examples in combat!" we shouted at combatants' funerals. Despite the undeniable truth of this slogan, it didn't completely dry the tears in our eyes.

In the hospital, as well as in the combat units, most people realized that, unfortunately, we were obliged to live surrounded by death, possibly even our own. Ours is a collective path; armed struggle was the ultimate measure we were forced to take to spare our loved ones, and all the people, from future suffering.

The civilians were also deeply convinced of the need for that struggle, and they, too, had paid a high price for it. But they lived more in harmony with nature, their labors following the seasons and the cycle of planting and harvesting. They bore children and maintained as normal a family life as the war allowed. Their arms for social change were the machete, literacy classes, and health education. In moments like these, the tragedy, the feelings of impotence and pain overwhelmed them. They were almost at the breaking point.

A *compa* approached me. "Can't you operate on Lidia, Paquito?"

"Why?" What could she mean, I wondered to myself? Lidia lay there on the porch, silent in death with the others.

"To take out the unborn infant, so God can welcome its little soul."

In three years of war, no other request wrenched me more than this one. Even though I don't believe in God, I couldn't bear her suffering so.

"Don't worry, *compa*. Things are in God's hands now. We don't have to worry about that."

I went back to the half-destroyed clinic. Orlando's neighbor Demetria and her weakened and emaciated mother, already over eighty years old, came to share their grief with me. The old woman lay down on the ground, refusing the stool I offered her. Ernesto, who died in the bombing raid, had been her only living son. While Demetria and I tried to overcome our shock by recounting the enemy's ruthlessness, tears ran down the aged mother's wrinkled face, dampening the Chalateco soil.

Then in the late afternoon, the people, some crying, others silent, filed up to the top of the hill to bury this day's dead. The bodies of the children rested next to their mothers in the common grave. Someone reminded the militiamen to protect the faces of the dead; one of them lowered himself into the pit and covered each head with pieces of rusty zinc, so the fallen would be recognizable at the Last Judgement.

The weeping grew louder; different songs were sung. Genaro shouted only once, "Revolution or Death!" and some of the people responded, "The triumph will be for the people in arms!" Then the men took shovels and machetes to fill the grave with dirt and complete this sad chapter of their lives.

In small groups, we slowly descended the hill. From the trail we could see the Sumpul, snaking in and out of the lush green lands below, lands which only the blood and the determination of the people have made it possible to control.

That night, guard duty was doubled in the event that the morning raid might have signalled an enemy invasion. When my turn came, I could still hear the rhythmic crunch of the millstones in the darkness as the women laboriously ground corn into flour, destined to be mixed with sugar as a food reserve in case of a *guinda*.

Melida's husband handed me one of the hamlet's two weapons. I checked to see if the rusty old rifle was loaded. If the enemy attacked, I was sure it would jam by the third or fourth shot. Was it for miserable weapons like this that these civilians were considered "belligerents," to be murdered in bombing raids like the one we had experienced that day in El Jicarito?

Even If We Have to Become Monkeys Again

It was the end of August 1984, and the crop was ripe in almost all the cornfields. In the hotter, low-lying areas of the controlled zones, the *compas* had already bent back the stalks, without breaking them off completely, so that as the corn finished maturing, it would be protected from the rains.

"That's the way we've always done it," one of the *compas* explained to me on the way to the orthopedic hospital.

That night a group of us gathered on a small porch outside the operating room. Longing to unwind a little, we chatted casually, sipping coffee and munching on sweet rolls, wishing time could stand still. I was on vacation and had returned to my second home to spend five days reading and relaxing—a real luxury under the circumstances.

I was in good company: in addition to Diana, there was Arturo, the head of the hospital; Federico, the visiting acupuncturist, and the two *compas* who had come with him. Federico told us about amazing enterprises undertaken by the Vietnamese that helped them defeat the Yankees in the south. They had billeted whole detachments underground and constructed subterranean hospitals, infrastructures demanding terrific discipline in order to avoid detection by the enemy. We felt deep admiration for this people, convinced that they had deserved to win. Yet, at the same time, we wondered how we would liberate ourselves if the Yankees did indeed invade us, since they were already so well-informed about guerrilla tactics. Suddenly it began to pour, a sweet and violent rain that brought us even closer together.

Through the torrents of water, we made out three figures approaching, wrapped in what appeared to be long cloaks, giving them a somewhat medieval appearance. As they drew nearer to greet us, in the yellow candle light, we recognized Evaristo, who at that time was the municipal political officer, and two other *compas* from the Subregional Government Council. They were thoroughly soaked, despite the plastic sheets they had held over their heads and shoulders.

"We've got an emergency on our hands. The enemy's broken through as far as El Tamarindo," Evaristo hurriedly announced.

"El Tamarindo!"

"And the hospital?"

"Information is sketchy, but it seems they were able to evacuate this afternoon. We were in a meeting in Conacaste when we got the news and they sent us to sound the alarm."

"Have you eaten, *compas?*" Arturo asked.

"Yes, thanks. We had supper in Huizúcar. We're off now to Patamera. We've got to warn everyone."

They said a hurried goodbye, and departed into the muddy, rainy night.

Arturo was an ex-combatant who, after having been disabled with a severe back wound, which partially damaged his spinal column, had become a lay nurse and anaesthetist. With the news of the enemy action, he immediately started with Diana on preparations for our departure the next morning. Our land mines and other defenses would prevent the enemy from advancing rapidly, so we judged that we still had that night to rest. However, as our little group went to sleep on the earthen floor of the porch, we worried about what tomorrow might hold in store for us.

At daybreak, the hospital became a noisy flurry of activity: wounds were dressed, emergency first aid kits were distributed, and medicine and surgical materials were quickly hidden in *tatus* along with the reserves of corn, beans, and other foodstuffs.

Messengers were sent to the Military School and the

PPLs asking them to send enough porters to transport the hospital's more than twenty bedridden patients. Since this was an orthopedic hospital, the majority of the patients couldn't walk. Diana took pains adjusting tractions, applying fresh casts, and immobilizing limbs with pins, in order to ensure that during the move, several weeks' treatment and immobilization wouldn't come undone.

Suddenly, several lay nurses from the El Tamarindo hospital appeared, followed by porters carrying patients in hammocks. Within a few minutes, the confusion that typically reigns over a hospital as it hastily prepares to evacuate was doubled by the arrival of yet another contingent of tired and hungry personnel and patients, already in retreat. The last person to arrive on the scene was Tomás, the head of the retreating facility. He was another ex-combatant turned lay nurse as a result of a wound—a lesion to a nerve in his right leg which still caused him to limp. Although he might never return to active combat, at least with a gun, there was no doubt about the strength and vitality of his commitment.

Somewhat overwhelmed by the confusion, we were nevertheless relieved to see all the *compas* safe and sound. They told us that they had been forced to evacuate in a tremendous hurry when the enemy took the hills above El Tamarindo, which overlooked the hospital.

During the past two years, the enemy had rarely invaded Chalatenango, and when it had, the offensives hadn't caused any significant damage. *Guindas* had become easygoing hikes, all but convincing us, despite the constant warnings from the command, that our territory was not only controlled but actually liberated.

Now Tomás was relating how the enemy, taking advantage of our inadequate surveillance, had penetrated as far as Las Flores, deep within the rear guard. Once there, they had launched a mortar attack, a tactic which typically precedes an infantry advance. The first projectile had fallen on the people's store in El Tamarindo, killing a baby girl, born only two weeks before to Irma, the shopkeeper. A spotter plane had then circled the area to detect movement and give a fix on houses and other targets. One of the *compa* radio operators intercepted an ominous enemy transmission from the pilot of the circling plane: "I've located the hospital. Send in the bombers."

On hearing that, the *compas* had immediately taken off, running to the hospital, which was a good twenty minutes outside the village, to sound the alarm. Simultaneously, word came that the enemy was taking the small chain of hills that divides El Tamarindo and Las Flores. The bombers could be there any minute, maybe even before the *compas* could reach the hospital. There was no time to lose.

But the hospital was alerted in time, and those who could walk had taken shelter in a nearby ravine. The critical patients were immediately transferred to the hospital trenches, while Tomás and Jaime went about preparing hammocks for them. Everyone spontaneously grabbed whatever materials seemed most appropriate. The lay nurses stuffed medical supplies into their knapsacks; Alex, the surgeon, loaded up the largest kit of surgical instruments, sufficient to perform abdominal surgery; Lisa, the anaesthetist from the National Resistance, one of the five parties in the FMLN, grabbed the ambu-bag and some pharmaceuticals essential for her work. Carlota, the cook, packed the sugar reserves.

Once the hammock patients were evacuated, two *compas* went back to the hospital and did their best to hide whatever materials remained. Since no one had anticipated such a full-scale invasion, the hospital was well stocked with impressive reserves of pharmaceuticals, surgical equipment, and intravenous fluid, far more than what daily or even weekly needs justified. There wasn't enough time to conceal everything in the hospital's *tatu*, which was now too far away anyway. So they just tossed everything into a hole created by a caved-in air raid shelter, then camouflaged the lot with branches and hoped that the enemy wouldn't find the stash. In addition to the medical material, in went all the corn and bean stocks, along with batteries, salt, and other supplies. There hadn't been any time for regrets.

Under the circumstances, the hospital staff couldn't count on the usual help from civilians to transport the wounded. The instant the people had realized the danger, they fled their houses, leaving their possessions behind. Although the hospital had several horses, these anemic, emaciated animals, covered with bites from blood-sucking bats, were out grazing in a far-off pasture at the time of the evacuation.

The less critical patients, including those with minor foot, leg, or head wounds, together with two *compas* who were recuperating from hernia operations, had no choice but to walk. Everyone on the staff took turns carrying the hammocks. Some lay nurses lasted no more than 600 feet before pleading to be relieved, or even worse, before dropping the hammock. That's how it had gone. Slowly but steadily, they had advanced along the muddy, rain-soaked paths, which became increasingly difficult in the growing darkness. Just before dawn, ten hours after leaving El Tamarindo, they finally reached the Sumpul river, normally just a two hour walk away. From there, local peasants had helped them make it the rest of the way to our orthopedic hospital.

Just about the same time as the arrival of everyone from the El Tamarindo Hospital, a platoon from the FAL unexpectedly arrived with wounded they had been carrying for over two weeks, all the way from the Para-Central Front, east of Felipe Peña. Despite the increasing confusion, we were glad to see the *compas* had arrived safely, especially since they had a radio, which we expected would make it easier for us to track the enemy's movements. From a hilltop, we immediately attempted to contact the Chiefs of Staff, but with no results. Hour after hour, the radio operator patiently tried to establish communication. Nothing.

Little did we know that, at that very moment, the Chiefs of Staff were racing down a gully, running for their lives. Without warning, the enemy had come within a few hundred yards of their camp. The *compas* detected them just in time, and had organized a hasty retreat, although typewriters and other valuable equipment had to be abandoned.

It was now obvious: our territory was being completely invaded.

Lacking further information, we decided to begin actually

evacuating the hospital. Just then we heard shooting nearby. A helicopter made an overhead pass, low enough for us to see the soldiers manning a machine gun through the open door. Fortunately, their fire wasn't aimed directly at us, but the sound of the engine and the shooting continued for some time.

Ten minutes after the noise died down, Blanca came running in with a couple of other *compas*.

"What are you doing still here? Don't you know that the enemy's just over in Huizúcar? They attacked a crowd of us with heavy fire as we were crossing the river there. We managed to escape because we were up front, but many couldn't get away. We're worried about what's happened to Jessica, María Chichilco, and Juana. They were in the thick of it with lots of others."

Everyone she named was important to us. Juana was the head of hospitals, while Jessica was in charge of the whole health sector, and María was a well-loved and respected party representative.

We were hard hit by this news, yet we had to finish packing and hiding the last of the supplies. All the while, we wanted to hope that the women hadn't been killed. Surely, some twist of fate had allowed them to escape. A hollow feeling, a horrible, sad tenderness overcame us. But this was no time for speculating. We had to get our people to safety.

I fetched my knapsack as the last group of patients was leaving. Among those fleeing was Virginia, a nine-year-old girl suffering from third degree malnutrition who had come to Chalatenango from the Felipe Peña Front with her mother and many other civilians in search of a more peaceful life. Her bloated legs were covered with sores. She was filthy and dressed in grimy old clothes. The staff had never succeeded in getting her to bathe herself or to allow us to do it, despite all our insistence.

Crying softly to herself, she walked slowly on her painfully distorted feet. Why hadn't she been evacuated with the first group? Clearly someone should be looking after her, I thought, but when Arturo ordered me to take care of her, I wanted to hide. Yet I knew his command was only right, and I couldn't get out of it.

"Come on, Virginia," I said, reluctantly giving her my hand.

She painfully walked a few more steps, still whimpering. I knew we would never get anywhere like that, so I grabbed her by the waist, hoisted her onto my shoulders, and hurried to catch up with the others.

I could smell the rancid odor of dried urine coming from her and feel her mucky grime sticking to my neck. The rejection and repulsion this little girl brought out in me made me feel like a real son of a bitch, but her slippery filthy hands were in my hair and on my forehead, and the stench was awful! Luckily, we were going downhill. I tried rationalizing my feelings, telling myself that my people were well-educated and overfed, and this was a way of repaying just a fraction of my debt to the hungry of this world. This thought eventually helped alleviate some of my disgust, but by then she was starting to get heavy. Although she appeared to be nothing more than a bag of bones, it was amazing how much all that water in her bloated body made her weigh.

Our disciplined column of hobblers, wounded, and porters was now climbing a steep slope, which offered no more protection than high grass and a few scattered trees. We eventually reached a relatively intact little house and were met there by Guillermo, a tall, broad-shouldered man wearing a wide-brimmed leather hat. I followed him along with the least operative of the group, those who couldn't walk, while the rest went on in search of refuge in a different direction. The burden of Virginia, meanwhile, had been assumed by another *compa*.

It was now getting late. Night was creeping over us as we made our way along the difficult path. Fortunately, Guillermo knew the terrain like the back of his hand. He proudly told us how, during the first years of the war, he had fixed up several caves for just this kind of emergency.

"You'll soon see just how nice I fixed up the one we're headed for," he commented proudly.

For the most part, caves had a bad reputation as shelters

since they were usually hot and uncomfortable, and water was always a problem. But Guillermo argued that this one was different because he had installed a bamboo pipe system which allowed air to circulate and prevented humidity from accumulating.

Finally we arrived. The mouth of the cave was so low that one of us had to crawl inside and drag the wounded in, one by one. Once in there however, we had enough space to stand in. The cavern even had a second floor, a loft constructed out of bamboo poles. Unfortunately, the structure had begun to rot in the humidity and was now about to topple over. There were forty of us in all, and still there was room for more. As our eyes adjusted to the darkness, we made out the forms of big containers of water, drawn from a nearby creek. What a relief not to have to go thirsty all night!

As soon as we got settled, the *compas* from El Tamarindo huddled together in little groups and went directly to sleep. The rest of us got busy organizing guard duty, which I was particularly interested in, since I was beginning to feel a burning fear inside me. If the enemy discovered us, we would be caught like rats in a trap. One or two grenades through the mouth of the cave would be more than enough to kill us all. The enemy would have to be blind not to see our tracks in the brush, I worried. I was assigned to the fifth watch.

After that, I finally settled down for a few hours of sleep. It felt warm enough not to need a blanket. I awakened some hours later to the dripping sounds of rain. I didn't remember where I was at first and wondered how I was going to keep myself dry. As I began to feel the raindrops, it seeped into my consciousness that we were inside a cave. Were the walls leaking? I eventually realized that I wasn't feeling rain at all, but rather drops of condensation; forty people breathing in a confined space, added to the natural humidity of the cave, had caused big drops of moisture to fall. I moved my pack into a corner where it wouldn't get wet and went back to sleep.

When it was my turn to stand watch, I picked up my already loaded M-1 carbine. My partner had a G-3. Except for an M-16 that one of the sleeping *compas* had, that was the extent of our arms in the cave. We spent at least half our watch groping through the craggy darkness, looking for a spot that would allow us to observe several different points from which the enemy might try an approach. The search was reassuring for some odd reason and helped steady our nerves. Though we never did find a good lookout, the night passed quickly and uneventfully.

The following day we received good news: the enemy hadn't followed us. Instead, once they had crossed the river, they had turned their focus on another area. Hot, wet, and thirsty, we all crawled out of the cave, and in relief, sat down near the entrance. The patients feasted on tortillas and canned sardines, while we each took out our sugar and corn flour rations. I had seasoned mine with sesame seeds and instant coffee to make the meal more appetizing as well as more energizing.

We were informed that, although the enemy was retreating from our side of the Sumpul, it was only in order to intensify its invasion on the opposite bank. We still had no radio contact with the command. Arturo decided to regroup back at the little house and send a small party, including myself, back to the hospital to check out the situation.

We still knew nothing more about the *compas* who were reported missing after the attack on Huizúcar. It was surely they whom the enemy had been pursuing before retreating to the other side of the Sumpul. The stories of those who had escaped the attack didn't raise our hopes. The enemy had opened fire precisely when a mass of people had gathered on the suspension footbridge over the confluence of the Hualcinga and Sumpul rivers.

"With my own eyes I saw María and her husband go down. They were left bleeding right there on the bridge," someone said.

Some people despaired, but the majority of us rejected the rumors, waiting for confirmation. We were also worried now about a group of wounded *compas* who had been scheduled to be taken out of the Front for treatment in exchange for the release of captured enemy army officers on the same day the invasion began. The exchange was to include fifteen disabled *compas* from each front. Our contingent was to gather near El Zapotal, where the International Red Cross would then take them under its protection. What had happened to them?

The first person to come out of hiding and bring us some apparently reliable news was Reyes, a combatant we had operated on the year before. He had been on leave, visiting his family in El Tamarindo, and thus had gone on *guinda* with the civilians.

His version confirmed the rumors that lots of people had died in the turmoil at the bridge. His group escaped up along the Hualcinga river. Unfortunately, several hours later they ran into the soldiers again. Since he was the only person to be armed with a gun, he fell behind to cover their retreat. However, it wasn't long before he heard more shooting and a confusion of screaming voices. No doubt, his group had run into the enemy once more. There was no chance of survival for that defenseless group of women, children, and elderly people. In the end, all Reyes could hear were soldiers' voices. There wasn't anything else for him to do, except make a run for it. He was convinced that his own mother and sisters had died together with the others. His expression wasn't exactly sad; he just looked as if a light had gone out somewhere inside him. When he finished giving us his news, he withdrew to a nearby stone wall and sat there alone, quietly and impassively eating tortillas.

Soon, to our relief, Jezabel, the doctor at the recovery hospital, turned up with her husband, Simón. We listened eagerly to what had happened to them. The attack in Huizúcar had taken them, along with Juana and the others, by surprise. The gunfire was so fierce and their reaction so spontaneous that Jezabel and her husband fled, leaving behind their six-month-old son who, although they didn't know it at the time of telling, was later picked up by Juana. They were distraught, thinking about what might have become of their little Derruti.

That afternoon, we set out with a group of *compas* from the Military School to search for survivors. Before long we reached the recovery hospital, and from there, we entered the area where the attack had taken place. For several kilometers all we saw were the *compas'* tracks in the brush and the leftovers from places where the enemy had planned ambushes: empty meat and vegetable tins, the remains of canned fruit cocktail, and Libby's tomato juice, all compliments of the Yankees. It was obvious that the enemy had combed every square inch of the zone, making us doubt we'd find any survivors. Simón showed us some brambles where he and Jezabel had spent the first night in hiding, barely a few yards from an enemy guard. We found knapsacks scattered about which had been abandoned by the *compas* in their flight.

We divided into two groups to continue searching. At a crossing of the Hualcinga River, my group noticed pieces of cloth on the bank. Soon more pieces, stuck to a rock in the middle of the stream, caught our eye. Taking a closer look, in the dimming sunlight, what appeared to be a corpse was trapped in the strong currents. We grabbed sticks, to keep our balance in the rushing waters, and waded out to investigate further.

I don't want to talk much about that bloated, discolored body, already dead for several days and beginning to decompose. Eyeing it closely, but never actually touching it because of some irrational fear that overcame me, I distinguished a necklace made from unusual seeds. The beads reminded me of someone. But who? Was this the body of a fat person or just a bloated corpse? Once we had crossed the river, we continued with our search on the opposite bank.

My companions hadn't recognized the dead person either. But suddenly, in the falling darkness, the face of Irma came to mind, the shopkeeper in El Tamarindo who always wore a seed necklace. Poor Irma, I thought, first they murdered the baby that she had awaited so cheerfully, and then they killed her. When I used to go to buy sugar, or some bouillon cubes to dress up a poor man's soup, she would tell me how happy her little girl would be, growing up in an already liberated country.

We didn't know until much later that, if we had crossed a little farther up river, we would have found the bodies of some thirty more civilians from El Tamarindo.

Ours wasn't the only search party; other groups from the Military School were also making sweeps. The following day, they found Concha, the only survivor of Reyes' group. They brought her to the hospital for treatment. A bullet wound had created a recto-vaginal fistula, destroying the urethra as well—a really ugly wound with serious potential complications.

Little by little, people had begun coming back to the hospital. The ambulatory patients came back under their own power. Radio contact had been reestablished with the command. Things seemed to be getting back to normal.

At midday, Noé, one of our surgeons, and Juana came out of hiding with little Derruti and some other *compas*. What a relief! And they brought us good news: both María and Jessica had survived, too. In fact, hard as it was to believe, and despite erroneous versions of the incident, only one *compa* had been killed in the savage attack on the bridge itself. This was the first really encouraging news we had heard.

Noé was on his last legs. He told us that a few days before the *guinda*, while he was accompanying a seriously wounded patient across the Cerrón Grande Reservoir, their launch had capsized when a sudden storm blew up. His foot had got caught in the weave of the patient's hammock, and they went down together in the waters of the lake. The patient couldn't possibly save herself, and Noé had been on the verge of using his .45 pistol to kill her out of mercy and commit suicide himself, when his foot suddenly broke loose. When he had surfaced, he grabbed hold of some aquatic plants and managed to struggle to shore. By the end of the week, though, he had developed malaria and, as if that wasn't bad enough, he also started suffering from a diarrhea which was resistant to all treatment. By the time he reached us, he looked like a scarecrow. No wonder he was exhausted now.

The military situation was still precarious. We were more or less expecting the enemy to attack our side of the Sumpul, so we were awaiting orders from the *compas* at the Military School who were now in charge of the zone.

In the meantime, Concha obviously needed surgery. Despite grave misgivings on everyone else's part, Diana insisted on closing the fistula right away. The other doctors tried to convince her simply to administer strong doses of antibiotics until the military situation improved. Furthermore, Arturo, as head of the hospital, considered it inopportune to remove the necessary materials from the *tatus* yet. But there was no reasoning with Diana. We even tried telling her we wouldn't assist her in the operation, but she only retorted, "OK, then I'll do it alone!" We emphasized how critical the military situation was. But she again refuted our arguments saying, "My stepfather was a colonel and I never respected him. I've never bought that military line before and I'm not about to start now!"

Finally Arturo consented. Yet just when Lea, her favorite scrub nurse, and Arturo, now acting as anaesthetist, had everything ready to begin, we got word that the enemy had begun advancing in our direction.

"This will be quick. They can't move faster than it takes to sew up this vagina," Diana responded.

The operation wasn't quick, or easy. The tissues of Concha's vagina were badly destroyed. The surgery was further slowed because Arturo had decided to administer minimal doses of anaesthesia, thinking that it would help avoid complications during the retreat. However, the doses were too small and Concha became so restless that he finally had to put her into a deep sleep.

Meanwhile, the *compas* at the Military School had no idea that all this was going on. Whenever they issued orders to evacuate, they assumed that we were all ready to mobilize rapidly. They couldn't possibly imagine that their orders would be subject to the termination of a delicate operation and that our retreat would be seriously hampered by a heavily anaesthetized patient.

But that's exactly what happened. About an hour later, a messenger brought strict orders to withdraw immediately. The Atlacatl Battalion had attacked the bridge over the Sumpul and was crossing the river not far from us. For the time being, a platoon of inexperienced *compas* from the School was holding them off, slowing down their advance. But the enemy was probably no more than 40 minutes away.

Diana insisted that she only needed five more minutes to finish suturing. Mario, a doctor and self-appointed leader, shouted at her to get the patient out immediately, but she continued working, without even so much as glancing up at him.

As soon as she had finished, in no time flat, Diana peeled off her gloves, threw the bloodied equipment in her pack and slung it over her shoulder. Mario grabbed up the ambu-bag with his free hand, while in the other he held the walkie-talkie which was instructing him to move without further delay. The enemy was closing in fast.

Noé and I placed the heavily-drugged Concha on a stretcher, since there were no more hammocks to be had, and together we took off. It was a constant juggling act to keep our patient from sliding off. If I were given a choice, I would gladly carry a hammock ten kilometers anytime, before ever having to go one kilometer with such a stretcher.

When we reached a stream, we saw an 0-2 spotter plane, which launches rockets with great precision, circling menacingly above us. Ahead of us, we still had to climb one more treeless hill, which offered no protection other than high grass and small bushes. Suddenly, several A-37 bombers appeared overhead, too. All bunched together, our column made an easy target; however, we couldn't separate now because the movement would attract the planes' attention. All we could do was crouch down and try to conceal ourselves as best we could. Just as we were settling Concha in a protected spot under some brush, we noticed two other severely wounded *compas* in hammocks out in the open. They had been abandoned by their porters. Taking advantage of the planes' temporary absence, we ran to fetch them and hid them under some trees near the stream.

The long column of patients, personnel, and porters who had left the hospital before us was slowly creeping up the bald hill ahead of us. I was sure the planes would detect them, and us, too. "We're done for," I thought. I was so scared I could practically taste death. Norberto, one of the wounded *compas* who had been abandoned, when he saw how nervous I was, kept telling me, "Take it easy, man." He certainly didn't want me to run off and leave him behind a second time.

To our great relief, we soon noticed that the planes weren't focusing their attention on our area but had concentrated their attack on the other side of the hill. They began firing more or less at random at what they supposed were our positions, in order to ensure the advance of their infantry.

This gave us a chance to reorganize the march, but we now had two more hammocks to carry. Seeing a column of *compas* from the Military School approaching, I asked the chief if he would assign some men to us as porters. Just then the spotter plane circled overhead again, so we had to quickly crouch down once more.

After that danger had passed, I realized that the group from the School was moving out, which would leave us with nobody behind us now but the enemy. I pleaded with several *compas* to help us, but to no avail. When the tail end of the column came in sight, and I still didn't have any volunteers, I stopped the last six men.

"You guys are going to carry hammocks!" I ordered, but they only started making excuses. Without thinking twice, I pointed my carbine at them.

"You heard me! Carry!" I barked.

So they carried the hammocks along a dreadful, overgrown path, that hadn't been used since before the war. I had surprised even myself at my actions, but there really hadn't been any other recourse. I'd never used my gun like that before, and it was an humiliating experience for the *compas*. Angry and bitter, they marched in silence. I was eventually able to better the situation by talking to them and sharing the load as we went along. When we reached our destination, I apologized and thanked them profusely. The resentment soon disappeared.

After a fortunately uneventful night, we hid the severely wounded patients in a new cave. Then the rest of us walked another seven hours, until finally we reached a favorable vantage point, high on a ridge. As we marched, we crossed paths with several combat units. Former patients greeted us with a special camaraderie. This was our ragtag army, with confiscated weapons, a limited supply of unsophisticated radios, and non-matching uniforms. They would be walking all night to reach the other side of the subregion. From there, they would attack the enemy's rear lines. The *compas* appeared in high spirits and eager to take on the enemy. The governmental troops had undeniably taken us all by surprise, but we were confident that it would soon be a different story. The *compas'* determination filled us with pride and confidence.

The high ridge where we came to rest was teeming with people who had converged from all over the controlled zones: the local civilian population, who always knew the most strategic places for holing up during a retreat, and *compas* from Radio Farabundo Martí, the Military School, logistics, the explosives workshop, the film and propaganda unit, and several other work areas. There were groups from other FMLN organizations with bases in Chalate, too.

Each group settled into one or another of the ramshackled or semi-burned-out houses found there. Since the health sector was so numerous, we had to divide up, occupying several houses. If you didn't take the necessary precautions, you might find yourself with nowhere to sleep. My little group took over a sooty old kitchen, which had a lumpy floor full of stones and hundreds of fleas. The little monsters had a heyday with so many people to choose from. We ended up spending three nights there, piled up one on top of another.

Guindas are special times for comradeship. They're when we come closest to true communist behavior, despite the fact that necessity often tempted each of us to look out for his or her own interests. I'd wager, on one *guinda* or another, that we've all set aside something extra to eat secretly at night. But in the end, someone always finds you out, and you're left feeling ashamed, with your selfishness exposed.

The ideology that develops in a *guinda* forces you to share. It is the moment in guerrilla life when you're most conscious that survival is only possible by working collectively. Community is manifested in lots of ways: the organization of the retreat, the different columns assuming diverse responsibilities, commonly shared misery and hunger, and the very fact that some do the fighting so that others can get to safety. Nothing exists in and of itself, but rather, only as part of the whole.

Sharing becomes a strategy for survival. There is never enough for everyone on a *guinda*, or, for that matter, even in more peaceful times. One day you've got cigarettes and the others don't; the next time it's your shoes that are falling apart, and somebody else knows how to repair them. You learn to give whatever the others need without keeping score, just as they aren't running a tab on you either.

In the early morning, those who were really alert went out to look for food, and before long, returned with sacks of young corn that were then equitably distributed. In time, small groups of people with similar interests formed. But one quickly learns to be careful not to join a group of only city folk, because the peasants are the ones who know the most about how to find food!

In our dilapidated house, we prepared a community soup. Somebody salvaged an old cooking pot. Others brought in *ayote* squash with *malanga* roots and different edible leaves. We added a packet of dehydrated chicken soup that someone else found in the bottom of a knapsack. Even those who didn't contribute anything had only to hold out some sort of makeshift bowl and say "give me a little" to receive their portion.

In this festive atmosphere, hungry and unbathed but happy to be reunited in the big guerrilla family, we held "seminars." The topics ranged from the Mayans to world politics, from art to international cuisine. Our group from the hospital visited with the other groups, too, taking the opportunity, for instance, to chat with the *compas* from Radio Farabundo Martí, whom we only saw on *guindas* since the location of their camp was a very well-kept secret.

The news was encouraging: the *compas* had maneuvered effectively behind enemy lines, striking at their weakest points without incurring a single casualty on our side. Upon intercepting the enemy radio, we heard its demoralized troops asking for food and women. The invasion had now lasted more than a week, and the soldiers weren't used to Chalatenango's hills and downpours. We expected the *guinda* would soon be over.

But suddenly, the situation turned for the worse. Word

came that the enemy was moving in to surround us. We would have to leave by night in order to break the cordon.

"Break the cordon." These were powerful, almost mythical words. In all the important *guindas* from 1980 to 1982, cordons had been broken, but only at a high cost in casualties. With such disproportionate fighting power, civilian massacres and generalized terror were inevitable.

The expression on everyone's faces changed. We all showed our tension and anxiety. In just a few minutes, the sociable atmosphere had disappeared and the deep-seated fear, which had been under control, subliminated by the flurry of activities, blossomed violently. Fear seized my very being, too, and I asked myself over and over, "What am I doing here?" All I wanted, at that moment, was to escape from that mountaintop, and from El Salvador itself.

How could we break a cordon with a bunch of hobbling, vulnerable, wounded patients? How could we defend ourselves? I looked at my carbine with its mere thirty bullets; the G-3 and the M-16 had no more than two magazines each. It was ridiculous—we were going to be slaughtered. There was no doubt about it. How could we ever control our fear and panic, so that we wouldn't just run off, abandoning the slowest? I had no combat training whatsoever. How could we possibly survive if breaking a cordon implied not only bravery but agility as well?

I had already seen so many die. I had watched the almost cool manner in which the *compas* reacted to death, which for them had become a daily event. Violent death had become as much a part of our lives as a sunset is for a peasant, something barely even talked about anymore. And yet, I was paralyzed in fear of it. Under these circumstances, my death would be nothing more than casualty number nineteen, coming after eighteen and before twenty. What meaning would it have? What would it change? It would simply be the end of my life. That's all. My death, symbolizing nothing, would just be one more casualty, like so many others had been.

In my internal hysteria, when I thought "like so many others," I suddenly wondered why, in fact, I should be any different. Why was I attaching a special significance to my own death? It was terribly arrogant to have committed myself to this war without accepting the risk of dying anonymously like everyone else. In reality, what gave my life meaning was not my death but rather my choice to live out a certain degree of personal growth and to contribute to this struggle, this transformation of history. The conflict between individuality and collectivity suddenly seemed absurd; now, the individual was dissolved into the collective.

> I believe the world is beautiful
> and that poetry, like bread, is for everyone.
>
> And that my veins don't end in me
> but in the unanimous blood
> of those who struggle for life,
> love,
> little things,
> landscape and bread,
> the poetry of everyone.*

I realized I would have to force myself to slow down my pace, half-trotting alongside the wounded, and use my gun myself or give it to someone else who could use it better. I felt that was the only way we were ever going to get out of this shit. The FMLN slogan "Revolution or Death" now took on new dimensions, and a certain serenity and feeling of security entered me that would never abandon me from then on.

I guess we all have to go through moments like these, each in our own way, and perhaps even more than once. If you resist them, you can't maintain the calm, the courage, the discipline, and the will needed to survive and triumph.

At sundown, we fell in with our gear on our backs. We were informed that the cordon had not been completely closed yet. What a relief! But even so, strict discipline would be necessary in order to move around enemy positions.

As I'd noticed on previous *guindas*, the *compas* from Radio Farabundo Martí, whose code name then was "Las Peñas,"

---

*Reprinted with permission from Roque Dálton, "Like You," *Poemas Clandestinos-Clandestine Poems*, translated by Jack Hirshman and Eric Weaver (San Francisco: Solidarity Publications, 1983).

were walking around as in a daze. Messages passed along the column: "Las Peñas—report up front," or "Where are the guys from Las Peñas?" Right up until the last glow of the setting sun, the radio crew could be seen looking like a group of bespectacled, absent-minded professors, lost in the mountains, wandering up and down the column, until they finally fell into formation with the rest of us.

At last, we started to move out. Learning to walk at night is something that either you get right fast, or you fall flat on your face and break your ass until you do. You've got to have eyes in your feet in the pitch black night. You have to spot slippery rocks, deep mud and roots, or branches blocking the path. You've got to watch the person ahead of you closely, learning from his or her mistakes, mutterings, and bitchings.

Your shoes are so important, you'll do just about anything to protect them. If the rainy season hasn't already started, at the first river crossing you usually try to walk on the rocks. With a minor miracle, you can get across with no problems, but you're most likely to take a royal tumble, soaking your precious shoes. The trick after that is not to let your backpack get wet. But that first dowsing has an advantage. At least from then on, you're no longer worried about getting wet in the subsequent crossings.

Considering how dark it was that night, we walked long stretches at a relatively fast pace. Up and down the column, people kept whispering, "Pick it up, faster." When we reached a fork in the trail, the order was, "The last one in each group waits for the next in line." However, it wasn't long before word came for us to halt, because "Las Peñas are missing."

To a certain degree, the news was a relief since we could sit down for a while and rest from the weight of our packs. Some people even seized the chance to take a quick nap. Before long, the order was heard again: "Pick it up. Whoever falls behind, gets left behind!" But that threat was never carried out. Instead, we ended up waiting for Las Peñas, and everyone else, too.

The weight of our packs, the fatigue, the exhaustion, and the pain in our feet got worse and worse as we advanced. I don't know whether it was a virtue or a defect, but I frequently fell asleep standing up when the column stopped. The problem was my knees doubled up instantly, and I would fall on top of the person in front of me, who would then turn around and bitch, "Fuck, man! Hold yourself up!"

The tensest moment was when word ran down the column to maintain utmost silence: enemy positions were within a few short yards of our path. We advanced with extreme caution, aware of our vulnerability and, at the same time, conscious that our strength was in our discipline and our capacity to handle the situation. Although it's natural to be afraid at such a moment, there's a special feeling of strength and pride that comes from being on the people's side, poorly armed yet shrewd as foxes. And that's how we slipped right through the fingers of the Atlacatl Battalion.

Upon reaching another strategically positioned mountaintop a little before dawn, we could look back on where we'd come from. It had taken us almost twelve hours to cover a distance that in daylight could be done in half that time. We rested there all day, slumbering in the shelter of the brush.

In the evening, after many more hours of walking, we finally reached a town which the enemy had previously evacuated. We were greeted with chicken soup and fried rice, prepared by combatants who had been harassing the enemy behind its lines. As we ate, we saw the sky light up at the other end of the controlled zones, illuminated by brilliant white bengal flares, like huge spotlights. We listened to mortar fire, grenades, and enemy guns as they blindly sought to liquidate the guerrillas. Now, with our bellies full, our tension broke and we burst out in exuberant laughter, mocking their futile attempts.

The next day the enemy abandoned the zones. Despite the destruction, the savage massacre of thirty civilians, and the capture of another forty, they had been unable to break us up. They hadn't even managed to inflict a single casualty on our people's army.

We were soon given authorization to go to the hospital in El Tamarindo in order to recover anything of value that remained. We didn't seriously envision finding more than bits and pieces.

Upon arrival, at first glance, everything about the hospital seemed normal. But as we got closer and saw how vast the destruction was, we just laughed, out of our rage and sadness. The hut that housed the kitchen had been torn apart, the Vietnamese stove smashed to bits. The soldiers had piled all the *tapexcos* in the middle of the ward and set them on fire. The operating room looked like it had been hit by a hurricane, probably as a result of a grenade blast. The roofing tiles of the pavilions were in smithereens. They had scribbled the usual graffiti: "Faggots, all you can do is run away." Other scribblings were intended to demoralize us, asserting that our officers had their passports ready to get out of the country when we were defeated. Still others were written in the rudimentary English these Atlacatl Battalion soldiers had learned while being trained by U.S. advisers.

The hole where the *compas* had buried the hospital supplies was empty. There wasn't a trace of anything. What could they have done with all that material?

After surveying the destruction, we decided to have a look at the hamlet of El Tamarindo. It too was reduced to ruins. There we met up with a militiaman, Oscar.

"What did they do to the hospital? Is it badly damaged?" he asked us.

"Good old Atlacatl fashion, brother. They destroyed all the huts and stole the supplies."

"So, that's what they were doing. I saw them loading cargo on mules and taking it to the helicopters. I was perched up in a nearby tree, you see."

"You spent the *guinda* in a tree?"

"Well, most of it. I was working in the cornfield when it all started, and by the time I got back here, everyone was gone. The enemy was already blowing it up. Since I was alone, I knew I'd better fend for myself. So I climbed a mango tree to get out of sight, and from up there I watched everything."

"Shit, man. You sure are brave."

"Well, tree climbing's no worse than walking. Look, pal,

even if we have to become monkeys again, we'll do it. Whatever it takes, we're going to defeat those sons of bitches."

This is a Hospital?

Uriel was wounded in May 1983, while participating with his Vanguard Unit in the attack on a strategic enemy stronghold, the town of Cinquera, on the Felipe Peña Front. He was hit by a bullet that first destoyed his hip joint and then penetrated his abdomen, rupturing the small intestine seven times. After being transferred to Chalatenango, he eventually left the Front in September of 1984 as part of an exchange for government army officers who had been captured by the FMLN. In France, specialists implanted an artificial hip joint.

The first guerrilla hospital I ever saw was in Guazapa. I went there with some buddies. All we found was a ramshackle house with four empty *tapexcos* inside and just one *compa* who was wiped out by a real bad bout of malaria. The only supplies they had were chloroquin and some swabs. Well, we said to ourselves, so this is a hospital? The day we get hit bad, we're going to be in big trouble.

Well, I did end up getting hit, and bad. When I came to, I saw a whole column of wounded being transferred to Chalate, two on each horse, hammocks, and all that. Shit, I said to myself, they may be able to treat two or three, but never all of us. I thought there'd never be enough medicine in the hospital for me.

I'll bet you were pretty worried.

I took it more or less in stride, it kind of made me laugh. After all, my wound was slight.

You thought your wound was slight?

We were used to seeing these really ugly injuries that ripped whole legs off in seconds, so mine didn't seem like any big deal. It was simply a matter of an operation, I thought.

When we got to Chalate, the hospital at Tequeque
There were lots of *compas* with really ugly wou
surprised to see more doctors there than in Guazapa.
ber them all—Rómulo, Ismael, Reinaldo, and Caro

But I imagine it was mostly the lay nurses who took care o   . Did they seem competent?

They did a pretty good job for the most part. They did everything they could. But sometimes there were problems. A few of them fooled around too much. Once when I was in really bad pain, one of the lay nurses grabbed my leg to do some rehabilitation exercises. "Take it easy," I said. She and I were always joking around and everything was cool, but this time she said, "So, it hurts, does it?" and gave me a good yank. I let out a scream and hit her hand to make her lay off. That caused a big stink, the *compa* crying and all.

Didn't it make you nervous knowing that just a few months before those nurses hadn't ever left their homes and didn't know anything more than how to make tortillas?

Sure. Most of all when they gave us shots. Some of the guys said, "I'm not letting her give it to me. She can be really heavy-handed." But others were more understanding, "They're still learning. How else are they going to get it right if they don't practice on us? Just grin and bear it today, and maybe tomorrow they'll do it better."

Did you ever have the chance to be treated by Arturo?

Yeah. Almost everyone preferred him. Some of the lay nurses thought you had to be really rough to cleanse a wound properly. We said, "They don't know how much it hurts." Arturo was really patient though. He'd been there. He had a softer touch, like almost all those who had been wounded themselves.

Since you couldn't go back to combat, did you ever think of becoming a lay nurse yourself?

Well, I thought about it for a while. It would have been a way of staying with my buddies, but the fact of the matter is, I just didn't like health work. Above all, I thought I would constantly feel disappointed, watching other wounded guys recover and go back into combat, while I would still be there, stuck in the hospital. That's why I decided that the explosives workshop suited me better. One-legged Juan was already working there, and later, some other disabled combatants joined us.

Shit, with Juan, we got along really well. He was in charge of administration and really threw himself into his work. He rapped with the guys a lot, and always managed to bring up something serious, something political or educational to think about. He raised our morale, and didn't let us get down or brood over our handicaps. He was a real example, especially with his amputed leg and all. We felt if he could do it, why couldn't we? He was a great comrade, a really extraordinary person.

What were the guindas *like for someone disabled like you?*

While I was still bedridden, there was that big battle in La Montañona, in August of 1983. Things were really heavy. When they gave us the news I turned around to see the other *compas'* faces:

"There's a *guinda*!"

"Well, yeah, a *guinda*." They seemed almost matter of fact about it.

"But we can't walk. This is going to be a real bitch."

Did you feel like despairing?

Whenever we thought things were getting really tough and that the chances of getting out were slim, we just joked about it. We began messing around. "Just think what the *Guardias* are going to do to you if they capture you," and, by the end, we were all laughing.

But what worried us the most about a *guinda*, of course, was being so vulnerable, being wounded and without even a gun at our side. We knew if they captured us alive, they would torture the living hell out of us. Those bastards would make mincemeat of us.

Well, that *guinda* we got sent to a cave. We stayed in there for a whole week. There were sixty of us, between lay nurses, wounded, and others. We all came out with scabies that lasted a good month. The worst part was being stuck in such cramped quarters. Sixty people in one cave—the heat was unbearable, there was never enough water, the rock ceiling dripped constantly, and there was no way out as long as the invasion lasted. Just imagine an entire week with no daylight, nothing to eat, and that itching. It was almost enough to drive you crazy.

Didn't you all have flour or something else to eat?

We only had a pound of powdered milk each for the whole week. And water could only be fetched at night. We had a terrible food shortage just before that *guinda*. Supplies were so short that we had gone whole days without a bite to eat. There were no reserves.

By my second *guinda*, I was already working in explosives. We got sent to another cave, only this time we could make coffee, since this one was equipped with a kerosene stove, and there was water right nearby to wash with and prevent another attack of scabies.

You could walk by then?

Yes, with a walking stick I could hobble about 600 feet at a time.

The last *guinda* I went on, during August-September of 1984, I wouldn't hear of going to a cave. I figured I'd walk it, but in the end, I couldn't take it. So I told the *compas* to leave me behind and we could reunite when it was all over. I spent ten days there out in the open with nothing to eat, but this time I did carry a sawed-off G-3 rifle. I crossed a river and hid in a cornfield. On the third day, I met up with some militiamen and we spent the rest of the *guinda* together, playing with the enemy, outwitting them, making fun of them. Not really a bad time at all.

How did you happen to be included in the prisoner exchange?

When I got back to the explosives workshop, they told me about the exchange. "If you're lucky, if some *compas* who we haven't been able to contact because of the *guinda* don't show up, you'll go. But if we locate them, you stay here." I said to myself: Well, even if it's just a way to to get some free cigarettes, that's OK.

How did our hospitals compare in your eyes once you saw the modern one in France?

We just said to ourselves: Shit! About the only thing the

medical teams in Chalate can rely on is their desire to do something. But for the wounds we get there, the *compas* need a hell of a lot of medical equipment that they just don't have. But the truth is, they do everything they possibly can for us.

But I Never Lost Faith

As time went on, disabled combatants, unable to assume tasks which required mobility, became one of our biggest problems on the Front. Several of them, like Tomás and Arturo, had become lay nurses. Others found their place in the explosives workshop and in similar sedentary jobs. Isaias, for example, recuperated in the Military School, where the disabled worked on instruction and propaganda. But others, like Edwin, who still needed medical attention, had to spend several months in the recovery hospital that we laughingly named "B-52," before eventually being included in the same prisoner/wounded exchange as Uriel.

Both Isaias and Edwin were wounded in the first half of 1983 and, for two long years, accepted, with struggle, the challenge of being disabled on the Front.

Edwin, you suffered a fractured tibia and your wound didn't heal for months.

Yes, it only healed when Diana finally operated and extracted a piece of rotten bone. She then did a skin graft, which fortunately took.

But then the problem was the lack of a plate (for the osteosynthesis). There just weren't any for cases like my buddy Apache's and mine. That's why, without saying a word to anybody else, we went to the nearby weapons repair shop and made two plates. Diana had explained to us that the plate should have little holes where she could screw it to the bone. We made them like she described, but in the end they weren't good enough, and she said it would have been too risky to use them.

How long were you in a cast?

Over a year and a half. When the plaster deteriorated, the doctors would make another one. At first, the cast was up to my hip, but after about eight months, they cut it down to only knee-high. With that smaller one, I was sent to "B-52" in Huizúcar. In the meantime, I kept myself busy, getting to know the young women or looking for something to do. I made myself a pair of crutches from branches of sturdy wood that a buddy cut for me. Then I set about making another pair for One-legged Benito, so I wouldn't have to keep lending him mine. I also helped the lay nurses, preparing bandages, swabs, and stuff.

That's how you fell in love with Jacinta. And in "B-52," how did you keep busy?

I wove fishing nets, swam in the river, and weeded the vegetable patch. Most of us also twisted string to make hammocks. I even mended pants and made handbags and other such things on the sewing machine.

Did you feel useful or were you just passing time?

Sure I felt useful. The hammocks were destined for use in the hospital and the people's army. To that extent I was still working for the revolution. But there were days when I just didn't feel like working. I brooded over getting out of the Front, or what to do in case I couldn't leave. It bothered me that, in every invasion, I had to go on horseback slowing the others down and increasing the risk for them.

Isaias, Bernardo cited your wound as an example of a very serious case, on account of the damage done to the lung, the diaphragm, and the intestine, which was complicated by septic shock. Furthermore, a nerve lesion paralyzed your leg for a long time.

Yes. Nobody thought I would survive, but I pulled through OK. Then I had to grapple with the paralysis caused by a piece of shrapnel. The muscles in my thigh ended up in a state of atrophy, and my lower leg became real limp. At first, I couldn't walk or even move my foot or toes. But with the rehabilitation exercises, I started taking a few small steps on crutches. Two hundred, three hundred yards—every day a little more. In addition to the warm-up exercises that we had done in the battalion, I got the lay nurses to help me massage my leg.

Later on, I went to work in the Military School and began

to run, but my foot was still weak. Even a small stone would make me stumble and fall. But I was really bull-headed and never lost faith that I was going to walk well again. I was an instructor for the new enlistees, which made me feel useful, and at the same time, gave me a chance to build up my strength.

You never abandoned the idea of being a combatant again?

Never. When they killed those people in the Hualcinga River, I was sent with my platoon of enlistees to the bridge over the Sumpul to act as a containment force. We ended up having to beat the hell out of there, but I didn't lag behind. That's when they decided that I was strong enough to join a commando group operating in some heavily populated suburban districts.

In the school, were you familiar with the FAPL propaganda group's work?

Yes, I watched them work quite a lot. They were really good at propaganda. People really liked what they had to say, it was simple and understandable. They knew how to work with colors and everything. They designed one poster that went over big with the crowd. It was inspired from a combatant's own words: "It's not so much my courage, as it is everyone's willingness to struggle together." I remember another that was hung where the lay nurses prepared bandages, with a quote from Che that said, "Toughen ourselves, yes, but never lose our tenderness." When I was there almost the whole team was new and Esteban taught them enthusiastically. They even improvised printing techniques. Even though he was missing an arm, "El Chino" learned to cut paper and print posters with a makeshift lithograph press they had there.

Did you observe how they proceeded when someone had an idea?

Yes. Each person sat down separately to analyze, think, or draw. Later they got together again and showed each other their work. After a lot of debate, they synthesized the proposals and then got down to work on the poster.

Did they also discuss the presentation, the colors?

Sure. They talked until they reached a consensus. There was a real dynamic atmosphere in that crowd. In the evenings, they rapped a lot, or maybe Esteban read books which everyone later commented on. It was great visiting them. There was a lot of cohesion there.

The Battle of "Lightning"

For almost all of the three years during which I worked in the territory controlled by the FMLN, I was in the Sumpul Subregion. I spent most of my time visiting the communities between Los Ranchos and Arcatao, walking from Los Amates to La Montañona. This is the zone where political-military control is most consolidated, and the civilian population is openly organized in PPLs (Popular Power Committees), under the jurisdiction of the Subregional Government Council.

Broadening the picture a little, the outskirts of the area could be described as a belt of towns surrounding our deep rear guard. We would go there to buy necessary items which we couldn't produce. The relationship established with these towns was not merely economic, but political as well. In many places, there were clandestine militias that defended their population, together or apart from the rest of the revolutionary army. Despite this, the mayors of Nombre de Jesús, Dulce Nombre de María, La Laguna, and San Fernando, for example, were members of the Christian Democratic Party and, in a few cases, the ultra-right-wing party, ARENA.

The situation in these territories has changed significantly during the different phases of the war. In general, dual political power is maintained over these communities. Rigid conceptions of a war don't fit the reality. The road from Dulce Nombre to San Fernando provides a good example.

Guerrilla control of this zone does not hinder travel along this road. It is used daily by trucks with huge loads of pine lumber or by pick-ups full of merchandise and villagers commuting to and from San Salvador. No doubt, enemy collaborators or spies from the government Long Range Reconnaissance Patrols also use it, but nothing happens to them, as long as they aren't detected.

This dirt road was not always as heavily travelled as it is today. It had been abandoned for a long time when, at the end of August 1984, it was reopened in response to petitions from the townspeople of San Fernando. At that time, the FMLN and the government agreed that if the State would repair and maintain the road, the FMLN would not destroy it, as long as it wasn't used by military vehicles. The agreement has held.

Enemy troops do travel the road frequently, but only on foot. Soldiers are brought by truck to Dulce Nombre; however, in order to invade the controlled zones, they must walk days and nights until they are able to engage us in combat.

My transfer to this zone, the Mountain Subregion, brought me lots of changes. Everything seemed new and surprising. I was again hearing the sound of automobile traffic, after two and a half years of hardly seeing even a truck moving from afar. On the other hand, there were more chickens, cows, and pigs in the area than I had become used to. The mountains were higher and colder too. And I had gone from the deep rear guard to a zone where the control was more fluid, more clandestine.

It was mid-1985 and our activity there was basically that of guerrilla warfare: sabotage, harassment, hit-and-run ambushes. As the *compas* said, "We defeat their overwhelming force with our limited means; we depend on quality instead of quantity." This tactical approach resulted, among other things, in fewer casualties for us. It was a matter of becoming strong and agile in concentrating and dispersing our troops, of preparing for a long term war or even for a direct U.S. intervention.

It was in this context that I took on my new assignment: I was to be the anaesthetist of the zone, working in a highly mobile and operative Medical Surgical Unit. This MSU was made up of Noé, a surgeon, Eduardo, our chief, and some young women lay nurses, among them Dinora, who was to be trained as an anaesthetist. I would be working there just long enough for Dinora to feel at ease in her task.

We led an exhausting life, trekking from one place to

another to attend to the *compas*. One day we were ordered to report to a field hospital still under construction in its new, relatively permanent location. We were met by Tomás, who had just been named head of the health care sector in the subregion, and by the hospital's general practitioner, Jezabel.

"Have you heard that we're expecting a patient?" Tomás asked, almost immediately upon greeting us. "We were informed yesterday afternoon and were really nervous, since we're without a surgeon. Besides, you can hardly call this a hospital. Jezabel and I are doing our best to build it, but they still haven't sent us any lay nurses."

We weren't exactly expecting our arrival to coincide with an emergency, but Eduardo comforted him, "Well, don't worry. If the patient arrives, we're here now."

The encampment housed the supply division, in addition to the hospital, and was located on a hilltop below tall pines that filtered the light, creating a splendid airy atmosphere. The camp consisted of a kitchen dug into the slope, several grass huts, and a series of small caves covered with pine branches, which the *compas* had dug out to serve as dormitories for two or three people each. It was the dry season and an icy wind blew continuously. At night, it became so cold that the only place we could bear the temperature was inside these caves, clustered together in fraternal embraces and bundled up in layers of sweaters and shirts. When we went to sleep, we used every available towel and blanket to cover ourselves. Who would ever have imagined that we were in the tropics?

Since we were hungry on arrival, we rapidly made our way to the kitchen. As we sat on a log with our bowls of black bean soup, Noé, our surgeon, asked for more information about the would-be patient. There still wasn't any news.

"We've finished the walls of the operating room," explained Jezabel. "And a roof won't be necessary since it isn't raining, but we haven't even had the time to make an operating table yet."

She had barely finished the sentence when Rigo, the messenger boy, announced the expected patient's arrival.

"In a hammock?"

"Yes. He's critical."

The patient was a combatant, wounded by grenade shrapnel during a harassment action at some distant point in the subregion. Members of his own platoon had carried him all the way to the hospital and, by now, nearly thirty-six hours had passed. Although his real name was Daniel, his companions called him "Lightning," and they told us that he was a first class fighter, audacious and clever.

We took the young man's vital signs and Noé inspected the wound. A fragment had penetrated his abdomen. At a glance, one could see that he was dehydrated and in shock. This was indeed a critical case, even more so given our circumstances and, to make matters worse, we had no more than one liter of saline solution.

Noé addressed the *compas* who brought him: "Don't go, men. We're going to check your blood types to see if any of you can donate blood."

"But, *compa*, we've been carrying. . . ."

"I know, but we have no choice about it. We have to find several blood donors or the *compa* won't survive." It was the only way we had to supplant the lack of serum. Turning to Tomás and Jezabel, Noé added with a touch of irony, "Let's inaugurate your hospital!"

The operating room was nothing more than four walls made of branches and grass. After considerable difficulty in locating a vein, I started the patient on our only liter of fluid. Eduardo and Tomás set about building an operating table, leaving me a few planks which I could use for the anaesthesia materials. In no time, things were advanced enough to premedicate.

In our backpacks, we had carried an authentic, although limited, set of previously sterilized instruments for abdominal surgery, along with gloves and other necessary materials. Dinora and I had also carried with us the anaesthesia equipment: an ambu-bag, one lone endotrachial tube, a few nasogastric tubes, and the basic, indispensable pharmaceuticals. And thanks to the *compas*, we now also had a unit of blood.

Shortly, Noé began to operate, with Jezabel's assistance.

Eduardo stood by and observed, as part of his training as a surgeon's assistant. Silvia acted as scrub nurse, with help from Esmeralda and Lina. Dinora and I placed ourselves at the patient's head. This time, Dinora was to be the main anaesthetist, and I would follow her orders. We had never before reversed our roles. She tried to convince me right up to the last minute that we should work as we always had, but I refused. Her hand trembled as she administered the anaesthesia, but everything went well, and the operation proceeded normally.

As for Jezabel, she didn't know that this was to be her last training session in surgery. One month later, during a *guinda*, she would have to perform a similar operation—a resection of the small intestine—alone.

There were no major problems, although every now and then Noé barked at Silvia for mistaking a clamp or for not handing him the right thread. As he began to close the abdomen, he snapped at Dinora and me, "Relax that belly! I can't suture it!"

I was forced to take over then, since I hadn't yet taught Dinora how to administer muscle relaxants. We injected a minimal dose of succinylcholine, between five and seven milligrams, to avoid provoking respiratory failure, while we guaranteed good oxygenation with the ambu-bag. We wanted to avoid the risks involved in intubation. Thanks to the transfusions, the blood pressure remained steady. Everything went fine, the operation terminating quickly for our conditions, after about four hours.

The difficulties were to come later. We were going to need a lot of blood. Luckily, Daniel's blood type, B positive, was fairly common. We already had secured two units from his platoon buddies, and we could count on another since one of the lay nurses, Lina, had the same blood type. But this would only last through the middle of the following day. What would we do after that?

Any operation in the abdominal cavity produces a temporary intestinal paralysis. The patient can't ingest liquids or solids orally until intestinal transit is reestablished. Under normal circumstances, such a patient receives three liters a day of dextrose serum with different electrolytes. Laboratory analysis determines the electrolyte dosage. Vomit, gastric juices, urine, respiration, and exudation are taken into account to calculate hydric losses, which must be compensated. It was more or less within our means to evaluate these factors, even if it couldn't always be done with exactitude. But analyzing the concentration of electrolytes in the patient's blood was impossible. We didn't have a medical laboratory there or anywhere else in the controlled zones.

However, for the time being, our biggest worry was the lack of intravenous fluids. As always, this was one of the principal problems of our medical logistics. How could we keep our territories supplied with this voluminous, heavy, and rapidly-consumed item? If ten or fifteen liters got to the Front in a month, that was considered an excellent supply. But that was rarely the case. Just calculating three liters a day per serious patient, without even counting minor operations, which always required at least a half liter, it's obvious that we were permanently short of this vital liquid.

In some circumstances, like Juan's amputation, we solved the problem by using fresh coconut milk, which is similar in composition to human plasma. Since a single operation consumes about two liters—the contents of four to five coconuts—this isn't much problem. But to sustain a patient for three days, about twenty coconuts are necessary, and such an amount had always proved difficult to acquire. Unfortunately, we were in the mountains, not on the coast, surrounded mostly by pine trees, not coconut palms.

We had often debated how to solve this problem. I remember one conversation in "The Café" in the hospital at Tequeque. Carolina argued that if the peasants knew how to make moonshine, we should be able to do at least as well by distilling our own saline solution. One of the doctors, Mario, thought this idea ridiculous. "And the pyrogens? What kind of filter do you want to use for them? Cotton?" he taunted, unwilling even to try.

But before the year was out, we had already distilled our first batch of homemade saline solution, using a rudimentary cotton and gauze filter. Earlier, we had heard that IV fluid was already being produced on the Para-Central Front and we had sent Ana, a competent lay nurse, to learn the procedure. Upon her return, she and some *compas* from the explosives workshop had gotten to work building a still, just like those the peasants made to prepare booze, using copper tubing and fashioning recipient vessels with zinc salvaged from granary storage silos.

After making some adjustments in the lids of the recipients, we had been able to obtain liters upon liters of intravenous solution. The formula was nine grams per liter of noniodized salt, which we weighed on a makeshift scale.

Unfortunately, we soon came to realize that we had serious limitations, because we did not have enough glass bottles and rubber stoppers for our production. In addition, our intravenous solution lasted only about ten days before it developed strange particles that could be seen when held up to the light. Distilling IV fluid was indeed an exacting task. Nevertheless, our still had provided enough liquid for all the operations performed in three hospitals, as well as several MSU's, during the period of the full-scale attack on the El Paraíso garrison.

I'll confess that when we had started using this homemade serum, not knowing much yet about anaesthesia, I felt very uneasy with the responsibility for administering it. I remember that the first time I set a patient on this solution, it was almost too much for my nerves. All I had on hand to counteract a possible allergic reaction was a single 500mg vial of hydrocortisone, a drug which was always scarce for us. On that occasion, to make a trial, we administered the fluid as we did blood: a fast drip to begin with, then a cut-off to watch the patient's reaction. We were lucky: there was none and the patient showed no sign of problems.

Indeed, in three years, I only heard of one negative reaction in all the time we used our makeshift IV fluid. And that one reaction may well have been due to our use of disposable materials which we had to resterilize and reuse repeatedly, and not to the fluid itself.

But it was now Daniel's bad luck that because the homemade solution expired rapidly and transport was so difficult and slow, we hadn't brought any in yet from the Sumpul Subregion.

So, what could we do to solve the problem of our lack of intravenous fluids? The only solution that we saw was to send a note to Daniel's platoon chief, requesting more blood donors. At noon, ten volunteers arrived to be blood-typed. From them, we were able to extract four 500cc units of blood, asking for more volunteers the next day.

We were very impressed by these young people's willingness to donate blood, given that they could well be in combat in a few hours. Their cooperation was an indication of the high esteem they held for Lightning and evidence of the solidarity that had grown among the combatants.

Things hadn't always been so easy. When we had first started giving transfusions, it had been very difficult to get donors. People thought that giving blood was harmful to them. Once in El Tamarindo, a dangerously anemic woman, who had suffered frequent attacks of malaria, was brought in by her family. The doctor asked them not to leave, in case the patient would need blood. At that, they turned pale out of fear and disappeared on the double. The whole time that woman was hospitalized, she didn't receive a single visit.

People didn't believe us when we explained how the body quickly replaces blood that is extracted. No doubt this replacement might be slower than normal in such a poorly-nourished population, but we didn't consider this to be a serious problem. To combat skepticism, several of us in the medical staff publicly gave blood so that the people would gain sufficient confidence to cooperate. Gradually they were won over.

Among the combatants, giving a blood donation was a little easier since they learned to see it as another necessary sacrifice in order to triumph. Many previously held ideas are often changed by the experience of joining the popular army. Relationships between men and women and attitudes towards authority are among the things that get modified. In addition, bashfulness about one's body, a deeply-rooted sentiment in the peasantry, is generally overcome. In fact, giving blood stopped being taboo as a direct result of the socio-cultural upheaval of the people's war.

The first day of Daniel's recovery was relatively uneventful. He regained consciousness, and we talked a little, although he was really weak. Between the other team members and myself, we never left him alone. The second day, we continually listened with the stethoscope to the sounds in his belly. We were impatient for the intestinal transit to begin again, since giving him so many transfusions was making us nervous. "Do you feel a fart coming on?" we constantly asked him.

In addition to looking after him, the lay nurses regularly sterilized all the instruments and washed his blankets, which inevitably got soiled when there were problems with the catheter or the IV lines. Dinora was particularly attentive to details, and her overall interest was outstanding. She made the most of that time to learn to type blood and improve her understanding of the theory behind it.

Dinora had returned from the refugee camps just a year before. Not even sixteen yet, she was plump, with kinky hair which she kept carefully groomed. Sometimes, after studying anaesthesia for more than three hours straight, we would talk.

"You know, Paco, this work scares me," she'd say. "For one thing, there are all the problems involved, and the math. What if I have to revive someone? I don't think I could do it. But there is something else too."

"What's that?"

"It's that. . . . Well, I see you here, far from your family and I admire you a lot for that," she hesitated. "But I want to ask Eduardo permission to visit my grandma near Arcatao over Christmas. We are going to be very far away and I know that once I'm trained, you'll be going on to another assignment. And since they can't operate without an anaesthetist, there won't be any one else but me, right?"

I didn't know what to say. She was very young for so much responsibility and for such a demanding life.

"I also know that the *compas* need me and they can't take leave often either." There was a long pause before she continued. "I think what we need to do is win this war so that we can be with our families."

As Dinora and the rest of us tended to him, Daniel proved to be very alert and especially attentive to his belly. On several occasions, he called us, "Listen to me. I think I'm going to fart."

But it was still too soon; all we heard was silence. We started to worry. Such frequent transfusions were dangerous. Blood is not just liquid, but also contains cells which can overload the organism. Besides, it was almost inevitable that one unit or another would cause the allergic reaction we feared.

On the third day post-op, we noted that Lightning's state of consciousness, and the rhythm and pattern of his breathing, had changed. Noé attributed it to a lack of potassium. The patient wasn't receiving enough calories either, and he was becoming noticeably thinner. Who knows what the chemical composition of his blood was at this point. If we didn't manage to rectify his electrolytic imbalance, his life could slip through our hands. This same damn problem had already killed several *compas* on the verge of recovery.

But we didn't have any injectable potassium. We almost never did, and since nothing could be administered orally, we couldn't give him potassium-rich food either. Suddenly, Tomás recalled having seen a bottle of potassium in a *tatu*.

"Well, send for it right away," Noé exclaimed.

We became somewhat more hopeful, even though we thought it was probably oral potassium. While Tomás went on his mission, we continued brainstorming.

"I have a bit of a folksy proposal, but we're desperate enough to try almost anything, right? If it turns out to be oral potassium, let's give it to him anally. The rectum has tremendous capacity for absorption, and we could add rehydration salts at the same time."

Noé thought about it for a moment, before commenting hesitantly, "Maybe. But that will stimulate the intestinal transit which could. . . . No, that's okay. Let's give it a try. Those goddamn intestinal sutures better hold up, or else."

"In any case, we can give it to him little by little," added Jezabel.

When Tomás returned triumphantly with the bottle, it was indeed oral potassium. "Potassium chloride 60 ml" was all the label said.

"How many milli-equivalents can be in this shit?" asked Noé.

"Who knows. Give him half of it."

We prepared a packet of oral rehydration salts, mixing them with the potassium chloride and went ahead with it.

We feared that the solution would flow out of the rectum immediately, but it didn't. An hour later, we gave Daniel some more, and continued doing so throughout the morning. By noon he was noticeably better. Little by little, his respiration and state of consciousness improved. We felt more optimistic, so we listened to his abdomen again. Alas, still nothing but silence. We had already removed the venous catheter because we had tortured his arms enough, pricking them time and time again. Phlebitis had set in on one of them. The situation was touchy.

While waiting for results, we sat in the sun outside the "ward," enjoying the view of the lofty pines against the crystal, windblown sky. Suddenly Dinora called us excitedly.

We hurried inside and there we saw Daniel, his *tapexco* and blanket all covered in shit, wonderful shit. He was a little embarrassed but we consoled him with our joy. We cleaned everything up and promised him a bath, *atol*,* and anything else we could. Suddenly, he farted and exclaimed, "Fuck! Give me something—I feel like I have to take the biggest shit in the whole world!"

His intestines seemed to sing under the stethoscope. What a relief! What we heard proved to be not just an overload of liquid in the rectum but true intestinal movement.

Once everything was in order, with Daniel reinstated on his *tapexco*, Eduardo announced that the events called for a

---

*A traditional Central American warm drink, made from a small amount of flour cooked in sweetened water or milk.

celebration and, with that, he set off to buy sweet rolls. Three days a week, a pick-up truck went down the San Fernando-Dulce Nombre road, selling all kinds of cakes and other goodies.

While waiting for him to return, we relaxed in the late afternoon sun. But our peace was interrupted when an urgent message from the Subregional Command Post arrived for Eduardo. We speculated that it might be announcing the arrival of another patient.

In minutes, Eduardo returned with several bags of rolls.

"You sure bought a lot!"

"Just one bag. The other two were a present from the salesboy. He told me, 'If I didn't have a family, I'd be fighting alongside you.'"

We gave Eduardo the carefully folded, stapled note. After reading it, he announced, "We leave on a mission at dawn. They say we have to drop everything, they need us right away."

"Hot damn! A mission! It sure is lucky that note didn't arrive yesterday," exclaimed Noé, and he lay down again to look at the reddening sky through the majestic pines. "Today was our turn to win a fight—the battle of Lightning."

Freddy

It was late, after nine. When I lay down on the ground in the ward of the field hospital, I could hear Freddy's rapid, laborious breathing from the hammock above me. I fell asleep as soon as my head touched the notebooks I used as a pillow. It had been a long day of uninterrupted caring for a critical and problematic patient.

Just after ten, I was awakened by the voices of two doctors talking with the head of the hospital, trying to decipher the scribbled message, recently received from the Subregional Command Post.

"Paco, they've authorized us to take Freddy out of the Front. Start getting him ready. You're going with him."

After discussing the details, they went off to bed.

"Did you hear that, Freddy?"

"Yes," he responded in a weak voice.

So at about 1:30 A.M., four *compas* placed the wounded young combatant in a hammock. We then walked the short distance that separated our camp from the road that goes from San Fernando to Dulce Nombre. There, we loaded Freddy, hammock and all, into a Toyota jeep, confiscated a few weeks before from one of the regime's ministries. It was a squeeze to get us all in.

At first, Martín drove with the headlights on, since the hills were high enough to hide us from enemy positions. But once we reached the crest, he turned them off and we continued by moonlight, descending a long, winding dirt road. All along that steep, rocky track we saw the evidence of destruction: a destroyed hamlet here, a bunch of shattered houses there. Freddy was uncomfortable and groaned when the jeep bumped across the streambeds on the path. Only once did we break the silence with a quiet laugh, when we surprised a cow in the middle of the road. We were nearing a populated area.

We soon left Martín and the car behind. Two of the six *compas* in charge of carrying Freddy tied the hammock to a pine pole to continue transporting the boy, now by foot. For my part, I inflated the blood pressure cuff that was wrapped around a plastic bag of IV fluid, to create enough pressure for the vital fluid to continue to flow properly into his vein, despite the difficult conditions which this form of transport implied.

An hour later, we reached a ridge of pine-covered hills. The *compas* caught sight of a fire and thought they detected movement. We halted while they checked their weapons, and then two of them went ahead. They discovered nothing more than a smoldering fire in the pines that had been burning for hours on end, a yellow glow in the shadow of the moon.

A mild northern wind carried the odor of burning pine resin, a smell so familiar in the chilly mountains. The top branches of the pine trees hypnotically swept the night sky. In time the boy got really heavy, and the transverse bar, holding him suspended, bit fiercely into the collar bones of the porters. When one pair tired, another relieved them.

We came to a group of houses. Quique, the transport squad chief, sent two men ahead to wake the people and see if they would give us a hand. I gave Freddy something to drink, passing a straw through the weave of the hammock that was wrapped around him like a cocoon. The boy hadn't slept at all. All the bouncing around was murder on his broken ribs. I glanced at the bag that was supposed to collect whatever flowed from the urinary catheter. There were a few drops of rusty colored urine, nothing really.

The *compas* returned with the first volunteer, barefoot and still half-asleep. He peered into the hammock.

"It's just a kid! And he's on IV. The other day one came through here who was really in a bad way. Maybe he'd like a tortilla?"

Freddy's "no" was so weary that only I could hear him. I had spent the last ten days and nights at his side and had learned to interpret his monosyllables and his silences.

"How old are you?" the barefoot man asked.
"I don't know," Freddy whispered.

Another volunteer joined us, and we started the march again. Luckily, it was a gradual, downhill grade. The ferocious pole of the people's ambulance ground into the peasants' collar bones. The two traded off with the transport *compas*. We advanced rapidly, passing more houses, incorporating more volunteer porters. No one asked where we were going. The war is full of secrets and discretion.

To the west, the moon was setting and, in the mountain slopes, fire was devouring acres and acres of land—precious pines, maize plantations, brush, pasture grass, everything, leaving a black sooty trail that only the rocks and clay resisted. The fire was perhaps set by rockets from a Cessna A-37 or a Push and Pull 0-2, or maybe by enemy vandals trying to eliminate the guerrillas' protective blanket of vegetation. Its glow in the night was so striking that we almost forgot its sinister origin.

To the east, the sky began to brighten, outlining the peaks of the Honduran mountains, so full of the history of the Salvadoran people. We kept up a good pace and, by seven, we reached the outskirts of a town. At dawn, Freddy's combat unit had already occupied the main streets to guarantee our passage towards the deep rear guard. As we entered, old women and young girls were already in the street, stretching and twisting the shiny cream-colored fibers of the henequen plant, from which they make ropes and string. They watched the guerrilla boy pass by, some with pity in their eyes, others with fear.

"Good morning."
"Morning."

One old woman handed Freddy some bananas and offered us tortillas.

"Poor little thing. How old could he be?"
"I don't know," Freddy whispered once more.

Despite the fact that the only truck that could be found in town was headed out in the opposite direction, Quique started convincing the driver to give us a ride.

"We need your help. We've got a seriously wounded patient on our hands."

The man made excuses, saying that his motor was in bad shape and that he was in a hurry. The truck was loaded with fattened pigs to sell in Chalatenango. He didn't want to spend any more on gasoline. But Quique was persuasive and didn't let him get away with anything. Finally, the man agreed to give us a lift.

We hung Freddy in his hammock in the back of the truck, amid the stench of the pigs. The driver's assistant separated the protesting animals to make room for us. It wasn't the best place for Freddy to travel, being a potential source of infection, but time was getting very short. The urine bag still had no more than a few drops in it. We had to get there before the level of toxicity got too high.

The truck bumped along the poorly-maintained, rocky road, that several years before had been financed by the Yankees as part of a counter-insurgency project. The driver went slowly and carefully over the severely eroded surface, but despite his efforts, the truck pitched and lurched, jolting the hammock and making Freddy groan in pain. His eyes pleaded with me to get this over fast. I hated the boy's suffering and was overwhelmed by a rush of anger at the tyranny that forced us into this war.

At present, we were skirting the base of a big mountain, where brooks and streams abounded, cutting across our track. Along the moist banks, green gardens flourished, even though we were still in the dry season. Towering above us were high cliffs, where imposing *guanacaste* trees clung, displaying new leaves from the first showers. The sight of cashew and mango trees made me dream of the fruit juices I would make for Freddy as soon as we were deep in the rear guard. I was feeling more and more drowsy.

Coughing and chugging, the truck climbed to the top of a hill. Through the already hot morning light, I saw the cold hills where the young boy had been wounded. I wondered how Freddy's story would end. It had been on the 31st of March— the day of the elections, that farce imposed by the gringos. That day the governmental army had invaded San Fernando with helicopters and two infantry companies "to guarantee the electoral will of the people."

The *compas'* counterattack had been successful, despite the enemy bombing with Huey UH-1H's and A-37's, which had lasted more than an hour and a half. They had shot volleys of rockets and electronic machine guns had fired who knows how many thousands of bullets per minute. Nonetheless, with nothing more than their determination, their badly-shod feet, and their confiscated weapons, the guerrillas had put the two governmental companies on the run, forcing the enemy to flee into Honduras. In the bargain, they had confiscated an M-60 machine gun and other materiel.

When the battle was over, the medical post had received only three *compas* with minor wounds, and Freddy, with a bullet in his thorax. We had immediately installed a thoracic drainage for him with the simple but efficient means at our disposal. We then operated on him and gave him a blood transfusion. Everything went fine, until upon leaving the makeshift operating room, the boy went into shock. He ceased being able to urinate spontaneously. We had only one adult-sized urinary catheter, clearly too big for him. What could we do? We had already had bitter experience with other cases like this. Improvising, we cut off a piece of disposable IV line, inserting this poor substitute for a catheter with great difficulty.

"Shit, he's bleeding. There's nothing but clotted blood coming out."

At that we gave him steroids and furosemide and kept him under intensive care. Soon we had to repeat the torture session with the makeshift urinary catheter. We had to know whether or not his kidneys were functioning. Nothing came out. So what the hell was going on?

In the afternoon, the *compa* had regained consciousness. He talked with his fellow combatants who had come to visit him. His manner delighted them, and it was obvious that they were really fond of him. We had to catheterize him once again, this time with an appropriately sized catheter that had finally come in from logistics.

It was difficult, but we managed. Yet only 30cc's of urine, mixed with blood, flowed out. We began to feel really desperate.

That night, to protect Freddy from the cold, we had him sleep in the kitchen of a house some peasants had let us use as an operating room. The lay nurses covered him with blankets and sweaters for more warmth. He still wasn't urinating.

At dawn, we had moved with the troops to a high, freezing cold mountaintop, covered with magnificent pines, which stood under a crystal-clear sky. A commander, who was also a doctor, visited us and examined Freddy lovingly. He confirmed our treatment and lifted our spirits. There weren't any signs of intoxication yet.

But that afternoon, the mechanism that held the catheter in the bladder failed. We had no other option but to resterilize the catheter and insert it again. We fastened it with a single stitch of catgut suture to the foreskin of the boy's penis.

Freddy screamed, but he withstood the pain. We explained everything to him. He understood. A great trust had developed between us.

The next day, with Freddy in a hammock, we reached the subregional hospital, hidden in the brush.

It wasn't quite so cold now. Several days passed and the boy's overall condition appeared good, deceptively good. Freddy asked for a tortilla and ate hungrily. He even took a few steps on wobbly legs.

When I reported his progress, the doctor exclaimed, "I don't give a damn if he's walking. I want him to pee."

Every evening, we checked the urine bag, but there was never more than a cupful.

We raided *tatus* looking for the last vials of furosemide and steroids. We read and reread the only medical text on hand. We wracked our memories trying to recall where ampicillin is eliminated. What if we did a peritoneal dialysis? But forty-eight liters of special IV fluid are needed to perform that procedure. Where the hell could we get that much in a poor people's war? We were overcome by feelings of bitterness, desperation, pain. By now there was no other alternative but to get Freddy out of the Front. So we put the case before the command.

That is how I became my guerrilla brother's private nurse: bathing him, feeding him, torturing him with injections, zealously watching the thoracic drainage, washing out his bladder, carrying him when he needed to take a shit. The boy did his necessities lying on his side on the ground. His feces were very watery and yellow, a sign that his body was struggling to adapt itself. I did what I could to comfort him.

"How is it you joined up so young?"

"One day I got the urge."

"In combat, were you cautious or really crazy?"

"I was always careful. It's better that way."

He told me then about his family. His mother was a victim of the first massacre of women in Chalate. He had a brother in the Special Forces and a couple of sisters in enemy-controlled territories whom he hadn't seen for six years.

"Don't you remember our meeting before, Paco?"

"No."

"When the hospital was in Tequeque. You were going down to the swimming hole with Ovidio."

"Ah, you were the one. . . . No, I don't remember."

The day before this long journey to take Freddy out of the Front, he had started vomiting, a yellow mass like his feces. Was his liver failing too? What the hell was going on? We discussed his medication again. Now we stressed the urgency of the situation before the command.

"If I vomit, will that help me get rid of the poison that you talked about?"

"No, Freddy. Try not to vomit, it's bad for you."

How is he ever going to replace the salts he's losing? I thought to myself.

"But where's the water going if I'm not urinating?" he asked.

Now during one of the truck's lurches I noticed Freddy clutching a one colón note in his fist. I made a sign, asking him who had given it to him. He pointed to the driver's assistant, a humble man who hadn't said a word the whole trip. Each time a vehicle approached us, the driver renewed his hope of pawning us off on someone else. "My engine's no good," he grumbled despite evidence to the contrary. But the other trucks were also loaded with merchandise and people, and so he continued on.

We were finally nearing the end of that sadistic road. The mountains were misty by now from the muggy heat. My mind filled with dreams and illusions:

Freddy marching along with a Yankee-made M-16, now being used to liberate his people. Dressed in his guerrilla uniform: confiscated fatigue shirt, non-matching pants made in the people's tailor shop, cheap fake-leather shoes.

When the road came to an end and the truck could go no further, we continued on foot. The sun didn't show any compassion for those who had been up all night. A passing *compa* helped us carry our load. In the heat and exhaustion, I found myself remembering the sun dance of the Sioux Indians: facing the sun with leather thongs pierced through their chest muscles, they dance until the dried leather straps tear themselves free, ripping out human flesh. That is how the Sioux men thank women and Mother Earth who give them life.

The pine pole was demolishing the *compas'* collar bones.

At last, we trod safe, familiar soil, deep in the rear guard. It was like being home again. We spent the night in the first encampment we reached. By moonlight, we left again at four o'clock. Yesterday's team was relieved by militiamen, sent by the people's government to carry the hammock. We were going still deeper into our territory. The militiamen, cheerful despite the arduous task, joked and teased the first one that asked to be relieved of the weight. In the first village we passed through, the Atlacatl Battalion had left its distinctive marks of destruction. A lot more houses were destroyed than the last time I had been through.

The day was dawning as we crossed the green, transparent Sumpul waters, so refreshing to our feet. One of the militiamen carried a radio. A newscast reported the latest health bulletin on the recently-elected Brazilian president Tancredo Neves' condition: already five operations, pulmonary edema, and so on. The glaring contrast was too much. Why should your chances for living depend so much on where you are born? I felt bitter.

Freddy had grown noticeably worse. Since he started vomiting again, at two different times I had had to give him injections to stop it. This worried me, because I didn't want to add more toxins to his already overcharged system. The IV lines and the venous catheter clogged often, due to the difficult conditions of the transfer. Over and goddamn over I had to find a new vein. Freddy could hardly talk anymore. Or smile. His stomach was bloated, and he was breathing rapidly and laboriously. It was obvious that time was running out.

Freddy walks out to prepare the corn field, with his machete in hand. The heavy rains will come and he'll plant the corn. By harvest time, he'll already be back with his combat unit, doing his share in carrying the heavy M-60 machine gun. The fruit of his labor will be for the people who made such a tremendous effort to save his life. For him, wherever he goes, there'll always be a compa *who will offer him a bowl of* atol, *made from the sweet tender corn.*

The people's ambulance continued its painful march, now on the shoulders of a fresh new team of militiamen who volunteered in the hamlet where we rested from the midday heat. Among the porters was Freddy's father, as well as the hamlet's volunteer teacher and other villagers.

As we walked, his father related how the boy's mother had been murdered. He told us that Freddy was only thirteen years old and lots of other things that I would have liked to have heard. But between concern for the serum clogging and my weariness, I couldn't pay attention.

The teacher and his partner were a veritable V-8 engine as they carried their burden. Knees bent, back straight, half walking, half running, they were people accustomed to carrying the terrible weight of suffering.

At sundown, we had to climb a bitch of a hill, which took almost an hour of immense effort. Freddy was exhausted. So was I. The teacher took pity on me and carried my pack. Freddy was almost too weak to groan.

Thirty-five hours after leaving the other side of Chalatenango, we reached our destination. There, with details wrapped in military secret, we would arrange everything for Freddy to leave the Front and receive the necessary medical attention, which we couldn't provide. It was only a matter of waiting two more days, but I doubted now he would be able to hang on.

When we took Freddy out of his hammock, and stood him on his feet, he could no longer hold himself up. His legs were like rubber bands. Shit.

I hung my hammock next to him and slept, but with one eye open for Freddy. Out of my sleep I could hear him talking with his father, "At least I did something to avenge Mama."

By dawn, Freddy's condition had deteriorated notably. The clandestine network was already operating, trying to make the necessary connections. Hurry up! We were on a beautiful mountaintop with sapote, mango, and *matasano* trees shading the coffee fields. The air was fresher than in the valley we had left behind.

The cicadas had already begun their litany when we bathed Freddy in the patio. After the bath, I had to find another vein and bitched with frustration: there just weren't any left that hadn't been mutilated. Maybe the answer would come at midday. We waited.

"I'm going to die today. My stomach's so bloated."

"Are you afraid, Freddy?"

"No."

"Good. You are a brave guerrilla."

As the heat grew, the cicadas varied their tone and kept on ringing. When we put Freddy on the bedpan, his bloated body was as soft as rubber in the hot sun and his breathing had changed rhythm. We knew this development was critical. We readjusted the IV.

We waited.
And waited.

Pains and spasms now invaded his body. We tried in vain to make the boy more comfortable, changing his position time and time again.

"Stretch my foot. . . . My hand. . . . Hold my hand. . . . My prick itches. . . . Take that tube out! Take it out! Oh! Oh!"

He stared at us for a moment.

"Go away. I want to die alone. Leave me alone."

Why did we stay?

The cicadas continued their indifferent litany.

"Stand me up. . . . Stand me up. . . . *Stand me up!* I want to get up! Paco, you son of a bitch! Stand me up! Stand. .me. .uu. . . ."

The cicadas shifted their tone again, but continued their insistent song.

"It was one of those impossible battles to win."

"Sure. That's how it is."

"What time is it?"

"Ten past four."

We're Staying Put

Demetria's house stood out from the others, not only because it had a cement floor and a tiled porch, but also because of the absence of harnesses, burlap sacks, and all the other odds and ends that are usually scattered around the porches of peasants' houses. Instead, there stood a rocking chair, a hammock, a big pine bench and, neatly stacked in the corner, a pile of carefully cut cooking wood.

Since the enemy had used this big adobe house as its command post during the November *guinda*, the house had remained intact. However, as a reminder of their stay, the *Guardia* had carved its initials, "G.N.," in big letters into the smooth finish of the porch wall.

For someone with the means to live a normal, even relatively comfortable life in another part of the country, it was truly extraordinary that Demetria stayed in the controlled zones. Yet there she was.

Although I often wondered why she'd remained, I had never asked her. I supposed her staying on was largely due to the powerful bonds that link peasants to their land. She and her husband had built their house years ago when they first came to these parts. And, of course, at the beginning of the 1980s, no one ever imagined that five years later the war would still be a daily reality. Hoping for eventual victory and peace, Demetria had stayed on and adapted herself to all the changes that the conflict had implied: shortages, suffering, *guindas*, danger, and the threat of death.

But there was surely another reason, too. In her own way, Demetria aspired to a better society. Although materially better-off than most, she was still illiterate and subject to an infinite number of beliefs and superstitions. She hadn't studied

Marx or Lenin, but she associated socialism with a more just system, with better education and health care for everyone. Her social consciousness was born, for the most part, of her Christian commitment. Close to where the National Guard had left its mark on the wall hung the only picture in the house: a portrait of Oscar Arnulfo Romero.

Demetria's family was also something special. Together with her lived Alba, her youngest daughter, who suffered from Down's syndrome, and Linda, her granddaughter, who was a deaf-mute. Martín, Linda's older brother, who was also a deaf-mute, frequently made the twenty-five minute walk from his house in a neighboring village to visit his grandmother.

The last member of this unique family was Demetria's half-brother, Andresito. Although he was not overly clever, I appreciated him as a quiet, simple man, and as a very hard worker. Despite a severe limp in his right leg, which resulted from a fall out of a mango tree when he was a child, he could cut and carry big loads of firewood and do all the other heavy tasks of peasant life. He spoke in a soft, almost effeminate tone. But in the evening, he liked to sit alone under the tamarind tree in the patio and sing *rancheras*, local country music, in a clear, strong voice. I often climbed the grassy hill that separated Demetria's house from El Jicarito to the sound of Andresito's solitary songs. His voice plunged me into yet another layer of bittersweet life in the Salvadoran countryside.

Demetria suffered from arthritis in her knees. Using a combination of her peasant science and my modern medicine, we tried every possible treatment: aspirin, anti-inflammatories, massages with kerosene or herbs, eliminating drinking water at night, and so on. We experimented with different diets: some recommended completely excluding hot peppers, while others called for large portions of garlic. Some of these cures worked for a while, and others didn't help at all. Despite all these measures, the pain in her knees increased markedly during the rainy season. So I sought Blanca's advice and we decided to put her on cortisone. Demetria began this new treatment at a very critical time: her brother, Ernesto, had just been killed in the bombing of El Jicarito. This personal tragedy was immediately followed by the stress of the August *guinda*.

As soon as the *guinda* was over, Blanca and I hurried off to see how things had gone for Demetria during the retreat. We found Andresito on the porch, sitting in the rocking chair, a homemade crutch at his side and one leg perched on a stool.

"What happened, *compa?*"

"I took a bad fall in the *guinda*."

Linda and Alba were thrilled to see us and ran to the kitchen to tell Demetria. She came out to greet us, but instead being of her usual serene self, she looked worried and anxious.

"Oh, *compas!* I'm so glad to see you! You wouldn't believe how upset I've been!"

Blanca examined Andresito's leg and found his knee very inflamed, but there was nothing that aspirin and a few days' rest wouldn't cure.

"In all the confusion of trying to get away, I tripped and fell. Just at that moment, a mortar shell exploded nearby. The pain was so intense I couldn't get up, even as more shells kept landing all around me. It was horrible."

"It's only thanks to the grace of God, and Orlando who carried him to safety, that he's alive at all," Demetria added in a sharp, nervous voice.

"Where was the enemy?"

"Right over there. That hill opposite us was just crawling with soldiers. We couldn't even grab the bare essentials. There was shrapnel buzzing everywhere. I really didn't think we'd ever get out alive. We fled all the way around to the other side of the mountain, walking all night. Look at how ugly my legs are from all the thorns and briars." Then she hesitated, embarrassed. "Heavens," she continued, "here I am carrying on when surely you're hungry. Let me fix some tortillas."

Once we settled down in the kitchen, Demetria's voice took on a more serious tone. "It's just not the same for me here any more. I'm thinking of going to Mesa Grande."*

Blanca and I were dumbstruck, dismayed. For us in the

---

*A refugee camp for Salvadorans in Western Honduras, some sixty kilometers from the border with Chalatenango.

war, it was always like a sacrilege, some kind of a defeat, when a *compa* abandoned the controlled zones.

"I'm over sixty now and I can't run around those hills like the others any more. If it were just me alone, I'd probably stay. But there's Alba, who won't walk when she's tired, and Andresito. On top of that, Martín and Linda are always running ahead of me and you can't call to them. They can't hear anything, you know. I just can't go on like this."

What could we say? There was no easy response to such weighty arguments.

Risking our lives everyday in this war had made us tough and demanding. It was true. We didn't want anyone to abandon us. But what could this old woman and her disabled family realistically do to defend themselves against the tyranny of the indiscriminate violence?

At last, Demetria broke the silence.

"What can I do? People are saying that the new enemy commander in Chalatenango has sworn he'll liquidate us all. The bombing of El Jicarito shows how determined he is to do just that."

"Well, that's what the enemy is planning. But don't forget that we'll be fighting back. Wait and see what's waiting for them the next time they try and come into our zones."

I was getting carried away with my own explanations until Demetria brought me back to reality.

"But what's going to happen to me the next time?"

"Why don't you build a *tatu*? I'm sure the militiamen and your nephews would help you."

"I already have one. But Chepe, who helped Ernesto build it, was captured. I'm afraid he might have told the enemy where it is."

Demetria put our tortillas on the kitchen table. Once she had served Andresito and the others, she came back and sat down with us again.

"To be honest with you, I haven't been myself since Ernesto died. I'm on edge all day long and I don't sleep well, either. Whenever I hear the planes at night, I jump up and run out of the house. Then I can't get back to sleep."

"But those are just spy planes, Demetria, not bombers."

"I know, but I can't help it. I just can't seem to find the sense of life anymore." She stopped talking and thought for a minute before asking, "Don't you have any medicine to make me sleep?"

We explained that it wasn't a good idea to get into the habit of taking sleeping pills. We tried to make her see that her sadness was perfectly normal under the circumstances, and that it was something which had to be lived through to be overcome.

"Perhaps you're right. Life teaches us that time heals all pain."

It was almost dark by now. Demetria lit a little homemade kerosene lamp. She went into the other room and came back with a small ball of wax and a wick she had braided herself. As we talked, she warmed the wax in her hands, stretching it, until she had formed a candle around the wick.

She liked telling stories, and we were interested in learning more about her life. She told us about how she had sheltered wounded guerrillas in her house during the first years of the war. She had nursed them and kept them hidden in a little room behind the kitchen. At night, a doctor would visit the house to make sure they were healing properly. But one afternoon, some National Guardsmen showed up. Demetria received them attentively, inviting them to sit in the kitchen where, within a few feet of the wounded *compas*, she entertained them with drinks and stories, until finally they got up and left.

"When the soldiers had gone, I went to check on the *compas*. With nothing more than a rusty old machete to defend themselves, they were very nervous. I told them not to fret—Demetria knew how to handle those bastards."

This storytelling was good for her and revived her spirits. But it was getting late, and we were all tired. There was only one bedroom in the house, so Blanca and I hung our hammocks alongside Demetria's bed.

Once I was lying comfortably in my hammock, I tuned into *The Voice of America*, since it was time for the jazz program.

"Is that music from your country, Paco?" Demetria asked from her bed.

"No. But in Europe we really like it, too. What about you? Do you like it?"

"Well, yes, it's different. But what I really like more is having you two come to visit and chat."

She blew out the candle, leaving Billy Holiday's melancholy voice to carry us away, each in our own thoughts.

Suddenly, we heard a mortar shell explode, and then another.

"Turn off the radio," said Blanca, agitated.

In no time, Demetria was at the door. There was another explosion.

"They're not falling near here. They're over by the Guayabo dam," Blanca observed.

In the direction of the hydroelectric plant, the sky glowed an intense white.

"Those are bengal flares. Perhaps the *compas* are harassing the garrison at the dam."

"But I can't hear any gun shots. Maybe the enemy's nervous and have frightened themselves again, firing at random into the night."

I was about to lie down again when Blanca told me that Demetria was crying inconsolably in the kitchen.

"It's odd that she's so sensitive. After all, this is nothing new for us," Blanca commented.

We wondered if her depression might be a side effect of the cortisone treatment and decided to give her diazepam for a few days. That night, Demetria slept fine and was delighted with the medicine. But in the morning, she looked worried and sad once more.

More than a month passed before we saw her again. As was customary during that period of the war, there had been yet another offensive.

Demetria didn't appear quite so frightened any more. Nevertheless, she told us she was still thinking about leaving. She knew I didn't like the idea, so she teased me and made jokes about going, toying with a brand new visor cap she had obtained for the long walk to the refugee camps. But suddenly, her tone changed.

"I still haven't decided. Do you think I could take life at Mesa Grande?"

"I don't know, but from what I've heard, I don't think you'd like it. You're used to your freedom here, even with the *guindas*. At Mesa Grande you'll have food and all that, but you won't be able to leave. And they say it's really cold there, too. But the most important question is: why go at all? In the camps, folks end up in despair because their lives are so restricted and sad."

"They say that you can return legally from there."

"But only to enemy zones. And now they're talking about making the people who return live in special camps, like prisoners in their own country."

I could see she was wavering. I really didn't know how I could help her.

Several weeks went by before I could visit her again. When she came out to greet me this time, I was immediately struck by how different she looked. Her characteristic self-confidence had finally returned.

"I've decided once and for all: I'm not going to Mesa Grande," she said triumphantly. I was pleasantly surprised by the determination in her voice.

"Yes, it's true. Mauricio came from Los Amates to visit, and we got to talking. Do you know what he told me? Well, he said that people here are watching me, waiting to see if I stay or leave. Everybody has reasons for going: children, parents, old people, the hardships, and the fear. Now that the invasions are so frequent, everyone is feeling vulnerable and wondering if life is still possible here. Mauricio says that every stone wall has a keystone on which all the others depend, and if you remove it, the whole wall tumbles down. Well, just imagine—he claims that around these parts, I'm the keystone," and she burst out laughing, amused at thinking of herself that way. "I don't know if what he said is true or not," she continued, "but it sure helped me make up my mind."

"That Mauricio certainly knows how to tell it right, doesn't he?" I commented.

"Indeed! Now I know that we all have a role to play here. Even if they kill us, this place is ours, and we're staying put."

Walking Salvadoran Soil Again: An Epilogue

> *For Ceci, youthful, talented, aware woman, peasant and lay nurse, killed in an ambush in March, 1987.*

Demetria wasn't the only one who had doubts about leaving. The hardships and dangers of the war made lots of people think about abandoning the zones controlled by the FMLN. Shortly after Demetria made her decision to stay, I found myself back in El Jicarito. Four or five of us were sitting on the porch at Melida's house, when once more the conversation turned to the same problem. But the atmosphere was not at all dramatic. On the contrary, we were laughing and making jokes about the situation. Melida, who with the help of her husband and eight children had rebuilt their house after the air raid, had the last word.

"Well, Paco, I believe you're one of those who won't leave. You're going to stay on with us," she said smiling, as she continued grinding corn on the millstone. "And you'll die right here in our land, just like the rest of us," she added with a hearty laugh that struck me as a bit strange.

A few days later, however, a message arrived ordering me to report to my base immediately. I was told that everything was ready for me to leave the Front. So I was going. I could practically taste the pizzas and fried chicken awaiting me. Yet at the same time, I couldn't help feeling angry about leaving my work unfinished, and sad to be parting with so many people I loved. Even so, I realized that after three years, it would be crazy to turn down this opportunity to rest, reflect, and see my family and friends again.

"We're grateful for your help, Paco. You know how important international solidarity is to us. We don't care where you come from, or what your background was. You've made a big contribution to our cause," Commander Douglas Santamaría told me in his farewell. And then, with surprising emotion for a man accustomed to the hardships of clandestine life and so many years of war, he added, "Don't forget us, Paco. Talk about us. Wherever you can, tell people who we are and why we struggle."

This wasn't the only time the Salvadorans had expressed their gratitude to me. Every time someone thanked me, I felt an embarrassed confusion, because I was not at all sure who had been helping whom. This book, more than a response to Commander Douglas's words, is an attempt to record everything that this dramatic walk alongside the Salvadoran people has meant to me.

Considering my background, it wasn't at all predictable that one day I would find myself sharing the anguish and adventures of a Central American liberation movement. I was born in the last throes of colonialism, a reality which I experienced directly. My parents were privileged representatives of the purest colonial style, well-to-do citizens from the mother country living in the colony. This was my everyday world. The residential neighborhood where I grew up reflected that reality.

However, just two blocks from my family home was the border with one of the city's vastest shantytowns. I looked upon the people living there with a mixture of suspicion and disdain. They were poor people, poor because they were incapable of taking initiative or of having the discipline necessary to improve their lot in life, or so the spirit of my education and upbringing taught me to believe. I belonged to an elite which felt itself destined to manage and control the future of the world.

Yet, as I grew, I found it difficult to comply with the rigid norms of that ruling society, so self-satisfied and convinced of its own virtue and glory. Rebellion emerges as a vital response which doesn't always have a logical explanation. The school I attended was a faithful reflection of my parents' principles and an effective transmitter of their society's values. But it proved to be intolerable for me. When I entered my teens, I finally left it and insisted on enrolling in the nearby public school, where the children of the more fortunate shantytown families studied.

At first, I didn't talk to anyone there, quite simply because I was frightened. Everything was so very different from anything I had ever known before. It was the other students who took the initiative towards friendship and, from that moment on, a whole new world opened up for me. They invited me to their houses and shared what little food they had with me. I got to know them and learned to understand what was motivating them and to appreciate their hopes for the future.

The struggle for independence was in the people's heart. Demonstrations and confrontations with the police were frequent. My new friends talked to me about their commitment to the cause, and they invited me to participate in their political activities. Even though I had never before expressed my rebellion in such terms, my classmates' frankness and generosity put an end to my initial hesitations. That intense personal experience made a big impression on me and, through it, I began to understand some of the reasons behind oppressed peoples' struggles all over the world.

When things in the colony started getting too tense, my father decided to return to the mother country. There, despite mistakes and detours, I never stopped searching. I joined different committees and groups dedicated to changing the unjust and alienated society, so void of any notions of solidarity, which I now lived in. We were constantly obliged to question the effectiveness of our actions, aware that we were up against a strong state that was as capable of total social control as it was prepared to coopt any true opposition. To a certain extent, we had success in our struggle, but it never seemed enough. Radical change was so far off, and my impatience to experience what a real revolution could be like grew stonger and stronger. All this eventually brought me to Central America.

Once in El Salvador, reality dealt me a startling blow. Bringing about revolutionary change was more difficult and so much slower than I had imagined. My romantic ideas of finding an enthusiastic collective of people, ever-willing to undertake great enterprises, clashed with the reality of working with specific individuals, with their varied personalities and different levels of political consciousness. I had to learn that a revolution in the making consists of small and very relative successes, of errors and partial failures as well. Nothing was gained effortlessly and there were no magic problem-solving formulas. Instead, the principal tools were constant, painful, arduous work, together with a discipline through which individuals exert themselves for the collective good. I came to understand that the revolution, the real revolution, is made up of lots of little revolutions.

As we worked together, the Salvadorans taught me many things. My collective experiences in Europe had little in common with the incomparably greater effort of living together and sharing in a *guinda*. I had considered myself a flexible and open person. Taking orders from a young, barely-literate peasant woman didn't pose any particular problem to me. That was something I could rationally accept. But when she criticized my impatience or dared to point out my lack of humility, I resisted strongly. Accepting such criticism was a much harder test than sharing housework. <u>I felt tremendous contradictions between my own needs and the collective needs</u>. Learning to submit myself to the group called for changes that proved difficult and disconcerting. That self-denial was a necessity wasn't easy to accept. The process was extremely hard, yet, finally, the very joys and hardships that I experienced, along with everyone else, brought me to work towards the unity in which many contradictions could be resolved.

Sharing the life of the oppressed is not only a rich experience, but a tremendous privilege as well. I learned to save lives in the worst possible conditions, to overcome hunger, thirst, and drowsiness in all kinds of situations. The tenacity and ingenuity we were all forced to develop became a treasure which cannot be destroyed by either the most sophisticated weapons or the comforts of an opulent society.

Life was intense there. There were precious moments of intimacy with the *compas,* as we huddled together, the rocky soil digging into our flesh, and formed a human wall of resistance against the icy wind that fiercely lashed against us. Today I can clearly recall the stories of peasants or youths from San Salvador about the humiliations they had suffered in the garrisons and the police headquarters, or in the streets. Their hopes for a new dawn for their children are still vivid to me. Under the stars, we shared our loves and frustrations, and our dreams of life after the victory. Experiences of such quality are difficult to repeat. When life is on the line everyday, men and women show what human beings are really made of.

Such living is not easily forgotten. Therefore, it should come as no surprise that, once again, I'm carrying my backpack full of medicine and walking the Salvadoran soil, this time with a greater sense of reality and a stronger dose of hope.

Subjective reasons are not enough to explain my participation and my return to the zones controlled by the FMLN. Without pretending to be a theoretician, I feel impelled to reflect on the why and wherefore of my presence, and that of other internationalists, in a war of such a national and popular character as that in El Salvador.

My answer will of necessity be somewhat personal and intuitive. Many people who have read this manuscript have commented on the importance I give the educational experiences in the war. The war is a school. That's how I see it, and that's how I experienced it, as both teacher and student.

The first time I had to administer anaesthesia to a patient, I didn't even know the correct dose. It was only later with the help of an experienced professional and comrade that I learned how to properly practice the essentials of this skill. After a year's work, I was able to teach the basic elements of this difficult technique to peasants who had only very elementary formal schooling, so that they could then function as anaesthetists in the hospitals and mobile medical units.

The same process occurred in my apprenticeship in internal medicine. I took on responsibilities at the outpatient consultation in the hospital in Tequeque, even though my experience in treating malaria, intestinal infections, or malnutrition was then nil. What's more, I knew very little about making a diagnosis. Yet, on many different occasions, I soon had to teach other *compas* what I had learned about these very same subjects.

Constant repetition of these educational experiences gave form and meaning to my presence in the war, not so much on account of their repetition, as due to my progressive understanding that, in this way, my participation was indeed efficient and truly satisfied a fundamental need.

The idea that I had formed of my possible contribution before entering the Front in no way matched the reality I ended up confronting. In my romantic, indeed, paternalistic vision, I imagined myself, deprived of medical facilities, single-handedly saving wounded *compas'* lives, relying on nothing more than my own wits and sacrifice. I never dreamed of meeting experienced doctors like Bernardo, who performed complicated operations assisted by teams of five or more. Nor did I ever imagine that the majority of my patients would be civilians. It never entered my mind that training others would become my most important job of all.

I can't emphasize this last point enough, since it seems to me it is more than just a subjective appreciation. I want to go beyond my own experience and reflect on the reasons that justify and even demand internationalist presence in El Salvador and anywhere else where people struggle for their liberation. Many of us, who come in solidarity from more developed countries, are insufficiently aware of the potential that our education and cultural background can offer, and of how useful such preparation can be in places like El Salvador. In a revolutionary struggle, sharing knowledge, helping to train others, and making up for the absence of educational tools become tasks that fulfill the passion for life and, at the same time, justify international presence.

I am discovering lots of changes on my return, little by little. Before entering the controlled zones, I spent several days in the capital, San Salvador. On March 24, 1987, seven years after the murder of Archbishop Oscar Arnulfo Romero, more than 60,000 workers marched under the banner of the National Union of Salvadoran Workers (UNTS). As I watched the demonstration from my hotel room, I realized that the popular movement had indeed grown. Just two years ago, it would have been unimaginable to put so many people in the streets.

Reaching the guerrilla camps had always been a risky venture. In the past, the journey could take up to several weeks. But this time, things were much easier. I walked from the last stop on an urban bus line to our first camp in little more than an hour. More than a mere anecdote, this incident reflects important advances in the guerrilla presence, in parts of the country that are theoretically under governmental control. Furthermore, it demonstrates a substantial improvement in the FMLN's organizational capacity.

On the way to the deep rear guard, I observed how much more extensive our control was over vast areas of Salvadoran countryside. The FMLN is now present in zones where its influence hadn't been felt before. Just walking along these very roads would have been sheer madness the first time I was here. Yet here I was, hiking along in broad daylight, wearing fatigues, and accompanied by *compas* armed with M-16 rifles.

The March 1987 attack on the El Paraíso garrison, resulting in its near complete destruction, was not an isolated action. Nor is the consolidation of a new war front, the Feliciano Ama Western Front, a fact that can be easily overlooked. The FMLN has altered its tactics. Its ability for rapid concentration and dispersion of forces has given the war a new face.

Everything is now organized on a smaller scale in order to permit greater mobility. Hospitals, too, have changed with this tactic. Two years ago, we had big "Guerrilla Hospital Complexes." Today, we operate in small units, distributed throughout the controlled zones. Each station consists of one or two doctors and half a dozen lay nurses.

It's not the novelty of the changes that I want to stress, but rather, their implications in terms of demonstrating the FMLN's capacity to adapt and to wage an effective war effort.

In addition to this, I have observed another relevant phenomenon: the repopulation of abandoned towns. Peasants once forced to leave everything behind, emigrating to refugee camps or to shantytowns in the capital, now enthusiastically welcome plans to return to their former homes and fields. Arcatao, Las Flores, Las Vueltas, and Tenancingo are examples of the firm decision of the people to make habitable, once again, the lands where they were born. Thousands have already gone back and are now living in these towns. They proudly regard their homecoming as a victory. They were fully aware of the hardships they would face. They well understood that their return to guerrilla-controlled territories would automatically make them become suspects, without any right to defend themselves. These villagers are still targets of an army that has shown no true sign of understanding the deep-seated drives and motivations of those who love life. In spite of this reality, these former refugees have chosen to live on their native soil. Their decision is noteworthy because it demonstrates a profound political maturity.

I don't want to sound too optimistic, nor indeed, to create false expectations. There is still no glimpse of a short-term solution to the conflict, and even less so, of an easy way to obtain it. But the false image so often offered in the media must be broken. The Salvadoran guerrillas have proven themselves to be much more than a condemned bunch of fanatics in a hopeless stuggle, out of touch with the population.

In the final analysis, my testimony boils down to a real and undeniable experience. What is occurring in El Salvador is a war fought by a people in search of liberation. More than anything else it is a people's war, a revolutionary struggle which has overwhelming popular support. Those who recognize it as such will understand what is happening and will comprehend the reasons behind this conflict, which has sustained itself despite all predictions to the contrary. Those who prefer to conceal the facts and formulate theories, more in keeping with their own desires, will be hard pressed to find explanations for the continuing vitality of this struggle.

When the objective of a struggle is the liberation of the

people, it is uncontainable. There will be more difficult moments, setbacks, and even momentary defeats. But history is on the side of the oppressed, and that is a powerful weapon. Revolutionary activity in El Salvador has persisted for too many years, against overwhelming odds, for the truly popular and just nature of this struggle not to be recognized.

For a Better Understanding of El Salvador: Further Reading

Literature

Argueta, Manlio. *One Day of Life.* Translated by Bill Brow. New York: Vintage, 1983.
A fictionalized account of peasant life, as seen by the women of one family, in the midst of the growing political struggle in El Salvador in the late 1970s.

Dalton, Roque. *Poems.* Translated by Richard Schaaf. Willimantic, Ct.: Curbstone Press, 1984.
A selection of verse by a major Salvadoran poet reflecting his preoccupations as an artist and revolutionary.

Dalton, Roque. *Poemas Clandestinos/Clandestine Poems.* Translated by Jack Hirschman and Eric Weaver. San Francisco: Solidarity Press, 1983.
A poet's voice among the guerrillas during the first years of the revolution.

Historical and Socio-Economical Studies

Anderson, Thomas. *Matanza: El Salvador's Communist Revolt of 1932.* Lincoln: University of Nebraska Press, 1971.
A conservative historical analysis of the 1932 popular uprising.

Armstrong, Robert and Janet Shenk. *El Salvador: The Face of Revolution.* Boston: South End Press, 1982.

A detailed history of El Salvador and its revolutionary struggle of the last fifty years, with special focus on the last fifteen years.

Bonner, Raymond. *Weakness and Deceit.* New York: Times Books, 1984.
An analysis of the U.S. role in El Salvador in recent years, written from the point of view of the former New York Times correspondent in San Salvador.

Brockman, James R. *The World Remains: A Life of Oscar Romero.* Maryknoll, N.Y.: Orbis, 1982.
A richly documented biography of a remarkable archbishop and his role in the Salvadoran political process.

Browning, David. *El Salvador: Landscape and Society.* Oxford: Claredon Press, 1971.
A highly reputed historical analysis of the problem of land tenancy and agricultural production in El Salvador.

Clements, Charles. *Witness to War.* New York: Bantam, 1984.
The author, a former U.S. pilot in Vietnam and medical doctor, relates his personal experiences in the Salvadoran people's war.

Dalton, Roque. *Miguel Mármol.* Translated by Kathleen Ross and Richard Schaaf. Willimantic, Ct.: Curbstone Press, 1987.
An account of the events of 1932 as seen by Mármol, a shoemaker, trade union leader, peasant organizer, and revolutionary.

Dunkerley, James. *The Long War.* London: Verso, 1985.
The story of the causes and the birth of the popular armed struggle and its development in the early years of the war.

LaFeber, Walter. *Inevitable Revolutions: The United States in Central America.* New York: W.W. Norton and Co., 1983.
An historical analysis of how economic and political dependency in the Central American region in this century has led to revolution.

Pearce, Jenny. *Promised Land: Peasant Rebellion in Chalatenango, El Salvador.* London: Latin America Bureau, 1986.
The recent history of the peasantry in Chalatenango, told from documents and from interviews made in the controlled zones.